The Locavore Way

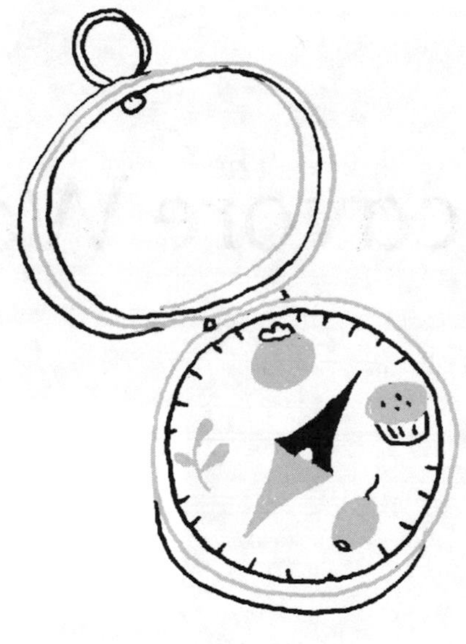

The Locavore Way

Discover and Enjoy the Pleasures of Locally Grown Food

AMY COTLER

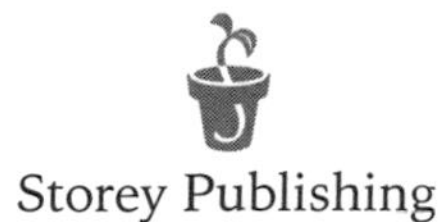

Storey Publishing

The mission of Storey Publishing is to serve our customers by publishing practical information that encourages personal independence in harmony with the environment.

Edited by Carleen Madigan
Art direction and book design by Dan O. Williams
Illustrations by © Marc Rosenthal
Indexed by Christine R. Lindemer, Boston Road Communications

Storey Publishing
210 MASS MoCA Way
North Adams, MA 01247
www.storey.com

Printed in the United States by Versa Press
10 9 8 7 6 5 4 3 2 1

Library of Congress Cataloging-in-Publication Data

Cotler, Amy.
The locavore way / by Amy Cotler.
p. cm.
Includes index.
ISBN 978-1-60342-453-0 (pbk. : alk. paper)
1. Food supply—United States. 2. Local foods.
3. Community-supported agriculture. 4. Farmers' markets.
5. Grocery shopping. I. Title.
HD9005.C67 2009
641.3'1—dc22

2009038244

Thanks

A special thanks to my husband and daughter, Tommy and Emma; to my sister, Joanna, for her editorial eye; to Cathy Roth, my local food companion; and to all the farmers who showed me the real thing firsthand. Thanks to my illustrator, Marc Rosenthal; to my art director, Dan Williams; and to my patient editor, Carleen Madigan.

Thanks, also, to those who lent a hand, sharing their expertise and trying out recipes, including Naomi Alson, Karen Arp-Sandel, Dan Barber, Amy Bodiker, Ellen Cotler, Ruth Dinerman, Rob Fairpoint, Elizabeth Keene, Robin Dropkin, Benno Friedman, Kathy Harrison, Melissa Kogut, Stacy Miller, Peter Platt, Judy Rabinowitz, Vikki Reed, Eileen Rosenthal, Kathy Ruhf, Jessica Savory, Rose Tannenbaum, Mark Winne, and Barbara Zheutlin.

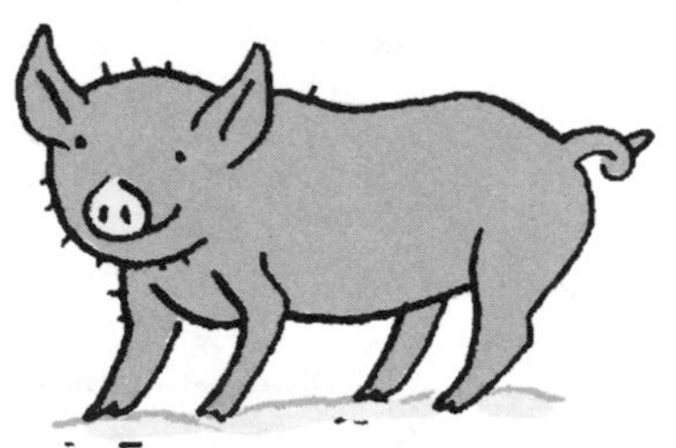

CONTENTS

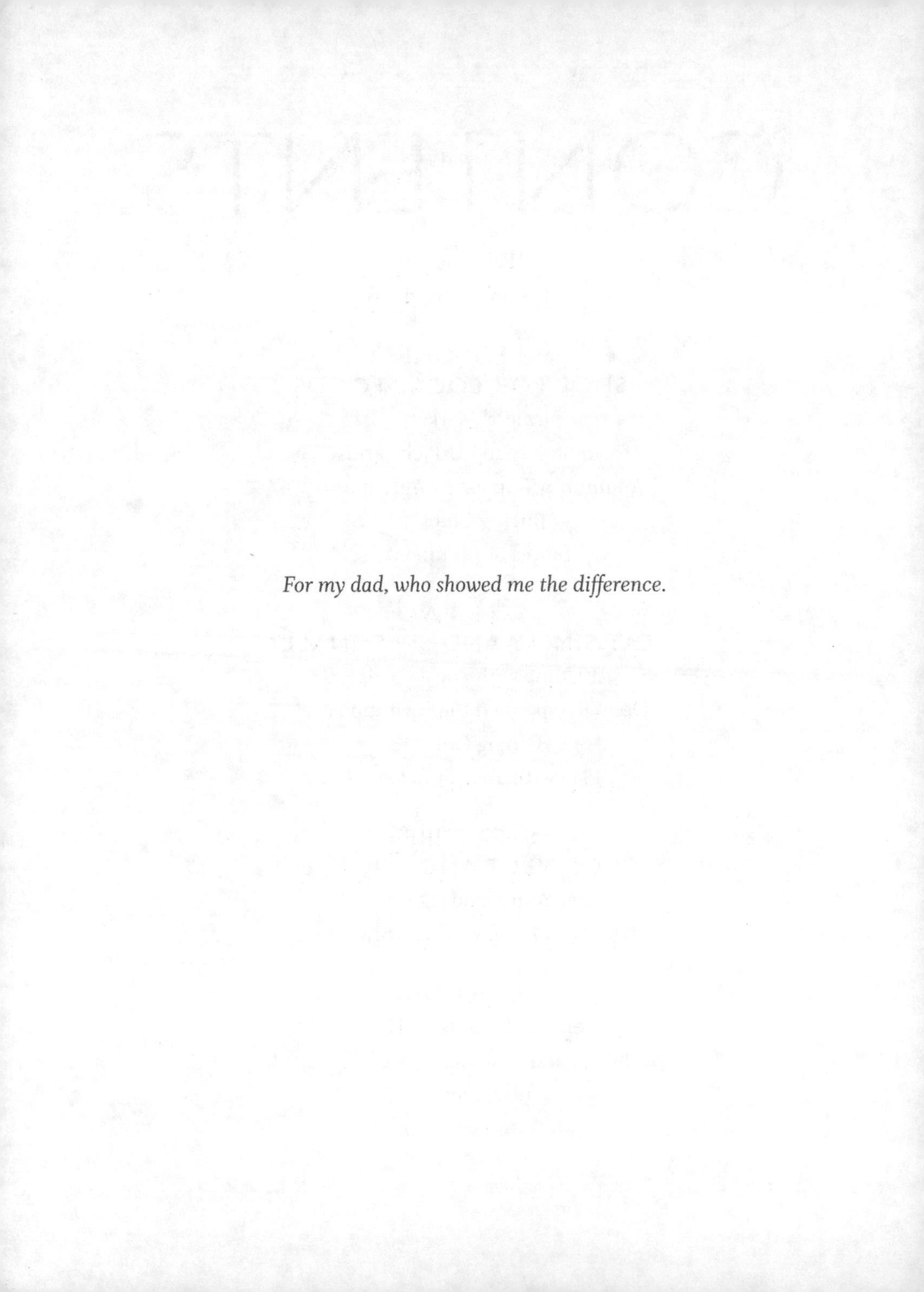

For my dad, who showed me the difference.

Locavore: *Anyone who seeks out and savors foods grown, raised, or produced close to home.*

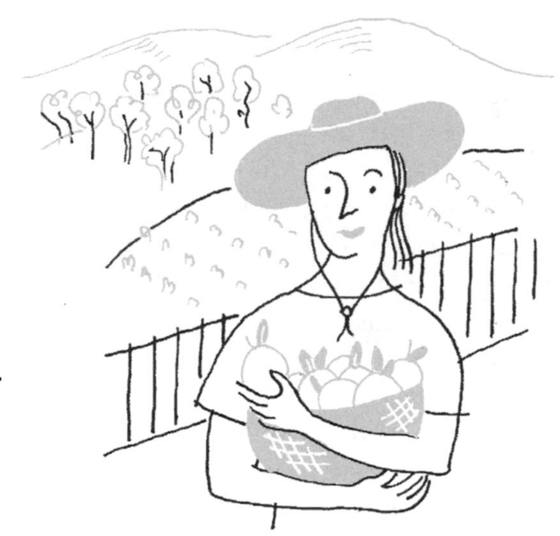

Welcome!

Bite into a Macoun apple, so tangy it cleans your teeth, handed to you at the farmers' market by Elizabeth Ryan, the farmer who grew it. Pick, then pop into your mouth, a raspberry — red-ripe and still warm from the sun — from Howden Farm, right down the road.

With pleasure and connection at its core, eating locally shifts how we engage with the most seminal ingredient in our lives: our food. The deceptively simple act of eating fresh, seasonal foods grown close to home is creating a wave of change. It moves us away from the horrors of industrialized farms and feedlots, with their seasonless foods produced for their high yield, low cost, and easy transport, toward something different: Imagine a healthy landscape, dotted with small farms raising food without ravaging the land, water, and air, promoting better-nourished communities and local economies, and creating less dependence on the fossil fuels needed to transport food from afar.

While the best part of eating locally is the food itself, its context and the stories behind it enrich the experience of eating it. The act of eating locally acknowledges agriculture's importance while encouraging farms to produce a multitude of distinctive foods, rather than the generic supermarket staples we see every day. And it provides a way for us to celebrate our diverse culinary traditions — together.

Let me be your guide to this new world of eating. As your local food companion — a pragmatic food zealot with 30 years in the culinary trenches— I'll show you how to plunge in, in your own way. I'll give you the tools for finding and sharing fresh local bounty, cooking and savoring it in season, and even growing a bit of your own food. There are numerous ways you can engage with your community to increase support for local food and local farms; I'll show you how to get started.

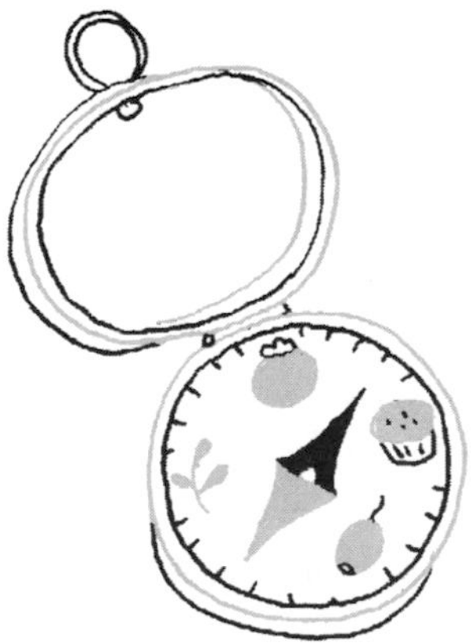

My goals are to respect your smarts, teach you how to make your own choices, then send you off into the world to change it, one delicious bite at a time.

MY JOURNEY?

I'm the lucky daughter of serious eaters. My dad fell in love with Japanese food as a code cracker in World War II. A Bronx boy, he grew beefsteak tomatoes in our suburban garden. My mom was a creative cook and hostess who had explosive culinary energy, cooking her way through Julia Child's endless cassoulet recipe and exotics like Indonesian Rijsttafe. This was balanced with typical Americana fare, like a dish that featured broccoli, fluffy white bread, and Cheez Whiz. They taught me to taste, cook, and seek culinary adventures.

When I was 7, we spent a long weekend in the Catskills on a family farm. There was a muddy pond, too many cow patties to avoid, and a goat who butted my little sister. But what I remember most was eating those eggy eggs — with their saturated, orange, stand-up yolks — in a sunny room overlooking the farm's beautiful fields, after having met the chickens, the farmer, and the farmer's wife (who had cooked the eggs). This was my first local food experience, and I was hooked.

Since that breakfast, many years ago, I've been seeking out farm-fresh food. And advocating for local farms and the foods they produce by encouraging connections between farms and consumers has become the core of my work. I was lucky enough to come of age during America's shift from the world of iceberg lettuce to a rainbow of salad greens. I've had the pleasure of working as a chef, caterer, educator, cookbook author, and food activist, all with the goal of bringing fresh food to as many people as possible, while empowering them to cook confidently with quality ingredients grown close to home.

My involvement with local food advocacy began when my family and I moved to the stunning Berkshire hills in western Massachusetts in 1990. By chance, I fell in with a band of heady agricultural progressives that included Robyn Van En, who spearheaded the groundbreaking community supported agriculture (CSA) movement in North America. The connection was transformative, bringing together the personal and the political, my passions for local food and for social justice. Through this grassroots group, which later became Berkshire Grown — one of the early local food and farms advocacy organizations in the country — I saw the farm-to-fork connection in a larger context. Our goal was to put a face on farming, on food produced with respect for people and the planet, to boost a localized alternative to industrial agriculture, as a means to literally eat our way to a better world.

Happily, since then, the local food movement has gone mainstream. Despite all odds, small family farms are emerging, fueled in part by enthusiasm over real food that's been grown well and by a backlash against poisonous factory farming. Although I've seen huge changes, it's still hard to buck a food system based on food from far afield. Now is the time to get smarter about where we take this local food movement as it grows and, in some cases, is absorbed by the larger system. I'm hoping you will join me on this challenging journey to create an alternative localized food system, using the actions described in this book, and eating blissfully along the way. Your path begins as mine did — with your first bite. This is *The Locavore Way.*

AMY COTLER

THE LOCAVORE WAY

15 WAYS TO BECOME A LOCAVORE

1 **Eat local foods in season.** They taste better. And if you want to go one step further, prolong the season by storing the harvest. How does raspberry sauce in the winter sound?

2 **Get out to a farm** whenever you can. It's where our food comes from!

3 **Buy fresh food directly from the farm** at a farmers' market, CSA, farm stand, or buying club (see pages 23, 40, 48, and 68).

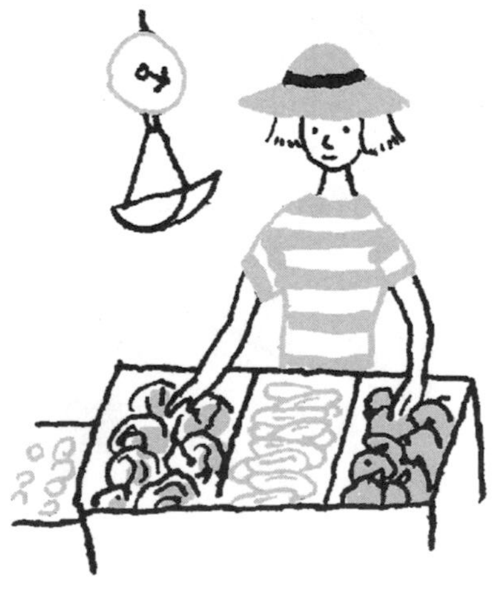

4 **Become a bounty hunter.** Track down local food in stores, from supermarkets to co-ops to mom-and-pop joints (see page 78).

5 **Feast on local food at home.** Cook more, and share it with your loved ones (see page 97).

6 **Have a party!** Make local food the center of holiday meals or entertaining of any kind. Include it at community events, fundraisers, and potlucks (see page 103).

7 **Engage the next generation.** Get out to the farm and pick your own produce, such as apples or cherries, with your kids. Bring local food into your child's classroom for a treat. Find out if your kid's school has a farm-to-school program. If so, boost it; if not, start one. Visit an on-site educational farm.

8 **Eat local food** in restaurants or anywhere you find it, like ice cream and hot dog stands (see page 134).

9 **Grow your own.** Start a vegetable garden in your yard, on your rooftop, or in your windowsill. Join (or start) a community garden. Garden

organically with diverse cultivars and promote a clean environment. Preserve extras for the dormant season or give food away to those who need it.

10 **Start a farmers' market** if you don't have one; invigorate your community!

11 **Boost access to healthy local food for all** (food security) by giving local food to food pantries, supporting programs like inner-city community gardens, and much more (see page 198).

12 **Eat more veggies and less meat.** Around 18 percent of greenhouse gases are caused by meat production. Besides, veggies are good for you.

13 **Give local food gifts:** premade, like wine from your region, or homemade, like seasoned vinegar made from farmers' market herbs or jams from your own berries (see page 92).

14 **Become an agritourist.** When you travel, find a food or harvest festival. Eat lunch at a farmers' market. Visit an educational or historic farm. Pick your own berries one afternoon.

15 **Advocate for a just, sustainable, and equitable food system** in your town, region, the world. Local food for all! (See page 198.)

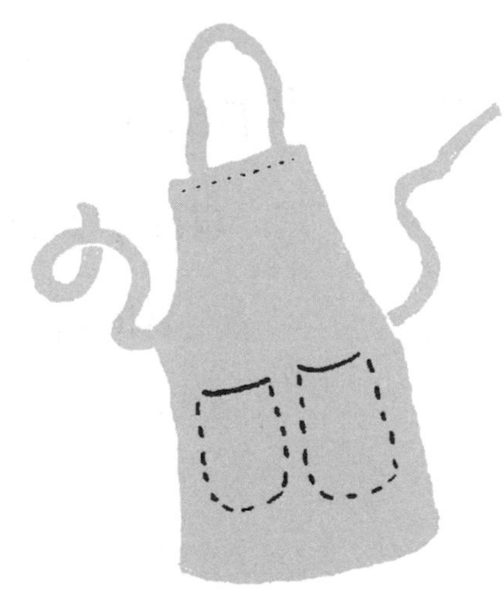

Getting Started

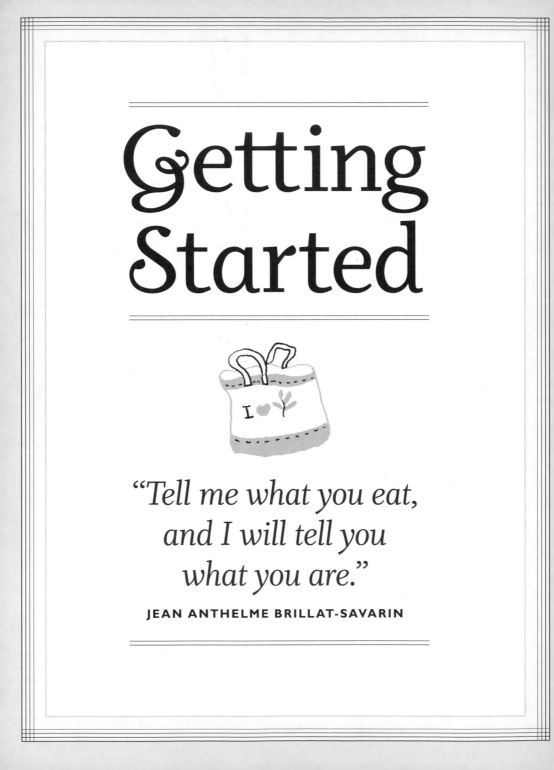

"Tell me what you eat, and I will tell you what you are."

JEAN ANTHELME BRILLAT-SAVARIN

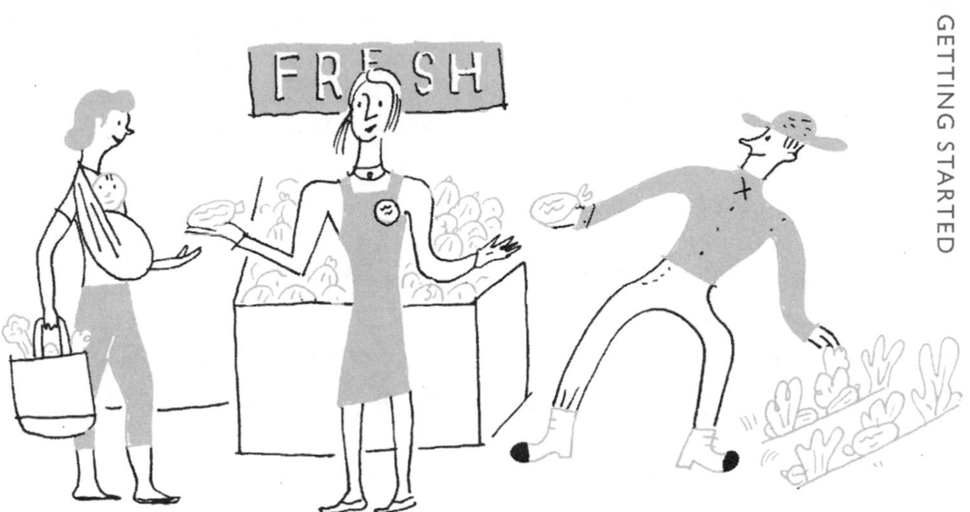

The Big Picture

Here's the crash course — what you need to know before we begin our local food journey. It starts with the basics about what local food actually is and why you should eat it. We'll unscramble tricky topics like organic versus local, emphasizing the importance of seeking out both ecofriendly and local foods. Then you'll get a jump start on becoming a seasonal eater, which is a central component of the locavore way. And finally, in keeping with hard times, we'll take a look at the elephant in the room — the cost of local food — and review some easy ways to cut costs before we launch into shopping.

WHAT'S "LOCAL," ANYWAY?

On average, your food travels at least 1,500 miles from farm to table. So how local is local food? When words get co-opted, they often lose their meaning, so I thought I should reinfuse the word *local* with the specific definition used in this book. **For the local food maven, the word *local* means as close to home (or wherever you are) as possible, and the closer the better.**

Local can mean picking an apple off the tree in your backyard, going down the road to a farmers' market, or buying food from 50, 100, or 200 miles away. A lot will depend on the availability of products, and that's determined largely by location and season.

Some people say that food from within 100 miles is local and anything beyond that is regional. I say, get as close to home as you can, and if that's regional, so be it.

IS LOCAL FOOD DIFFERENT?

Local food tends to be fresher, more distinctive in flavor, less generic. This is what the French call *terroir,* or "a taste of place." It's a term that is often associated with wine and cheese, but it's just as useful in describing other kinds of food, as well.

Local food is often, but not always, from small- and medium-sized farms, many of which are striving to bring you food that has been produced while replenishing — rather than depleting — our resources, land, and people. Those farms have also helped bring back some of the vast biodiversity of plant varieties and animal breeds essential to a robust environment (and a delicious diet). Local food carries its origins and context with it, and gives us more pleasure and better flavor as a result. It's different because of the way it bonds us to our families and friends, neighbors, community, and region, grounding us in what often seems a detached and fragmented world.

WHY BUY LOCALLY?

We all need to learn (or be reminded of) why we bother to eat locally grown, raised, and produced foods because, while the rewards are vast (and edible), procuring local food isn't always as easy as bopping over to the supermarket for a one-stop shop. So following are 10 reasons to integrate local foods into your life, whether it's including a Saturday-morning farmers' market outing in your weekend plans or swinging by an orchard to pick up fresh-pressed cider on your way home from work.

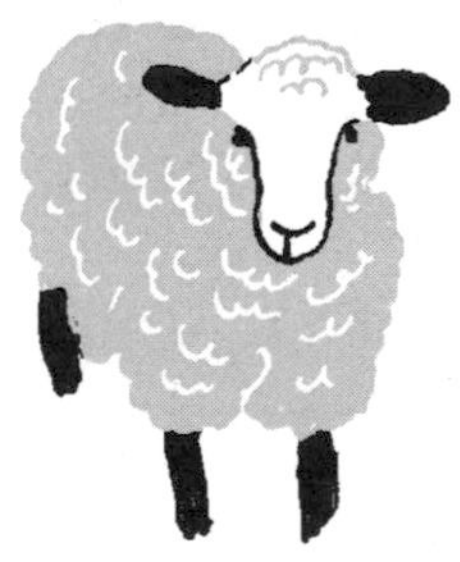

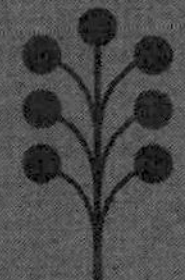

The Industrial Eater

"The industrial eater is, in fact, one who does not know that eating is an agricultural act, who no longer knows or imagines the connections between eating and the land, and who is therefore necessarily passive and uncritical. We still (sometimes) remember that we cannot be free if our minds and voices are controlled by someone else. But we have neglected to understand that we cannot be free if our food is controlled by someone else. The condition of the passive consumer of food is not a democratic condition. One reason to eat responsibly is to live free."

WENDELL BERRY

WHY BOTHER?

10 REASONS TO EAT LOCALLY PRODUCED FOOD

Each bite of food contains the world. Inside that crisp fall apple is the story of where, how, and by whom it was grown, harvested, and brought to us. And so we shape our world by what we eat.

1 **For the sheer pleasure of it.** Savor ultimate taste and freshness. You can't beat food that's been grown for its flavor rather than for its ability to be shipped long distances (or, in the case of animals, the ability to fatten up quickly). Finding and eating it, as well as growing and raising it, is a pleasure, whether you are biting into a juicy peach right from the tree or savoring a farmers' market meal with family and friends. It's not generic food; you can taste the life in it.

2 **To connect.** Connecting the dots from farm to table encourages us to bond with people and places. Get to know your farmer and fellow shoppers at the market. Share your bounty with friends, family, and community, especially those in need. Embrace nature as you follow the flow of the seasons through local food wherever you live.

3 **For the health and safety of your family and yourself.** Just-picked fresh local food is more nutritious than groceries sitting and aging on their shelves. Besides, local foods are often raised by sustainable practices, and that means you eat fewer harmful chemicals, breathe better air, and drink cleaner water. Access to food grown close to home is the ultimate homeland security.

What's the best food memory you have? Most likely it's about relationships as much as food — about love and connection.

All good food connects us, but local food goes one step further.

4 For the health of our planet. Eating local food, sustainably raised, promotes an ecofriendly food system. Conventionally raised food depletes the land, water, and air. Food grown close to home uses less fossil fuel to reach us, which means less pollution and less dependence on nonrenewable resources. Did you know that it takes ten calories of fossil fuel energy to produce one calorie of supermarket food?

5 To boost the local economy, community, and region. Local food dollars spent close to home sustain local economies with independently owned farms and other businesses. Ever go on a trip, only to spot the same strip of stores you have at home, all importing their products? Food dollars spent locally, on the other hand, are reinvested in the community, building relationships among people. Local food venues, especially farmers' markets, invigorate their communities, creating a vibrant hub, like a town green.

6 For an open, working landscape. Farms preserve our beautiful open, working landscape, a vital part of a healthy region with varied land use. Support for the harvesting of wild-crafted foods, such as wild rice, helps protect our natural habitats.

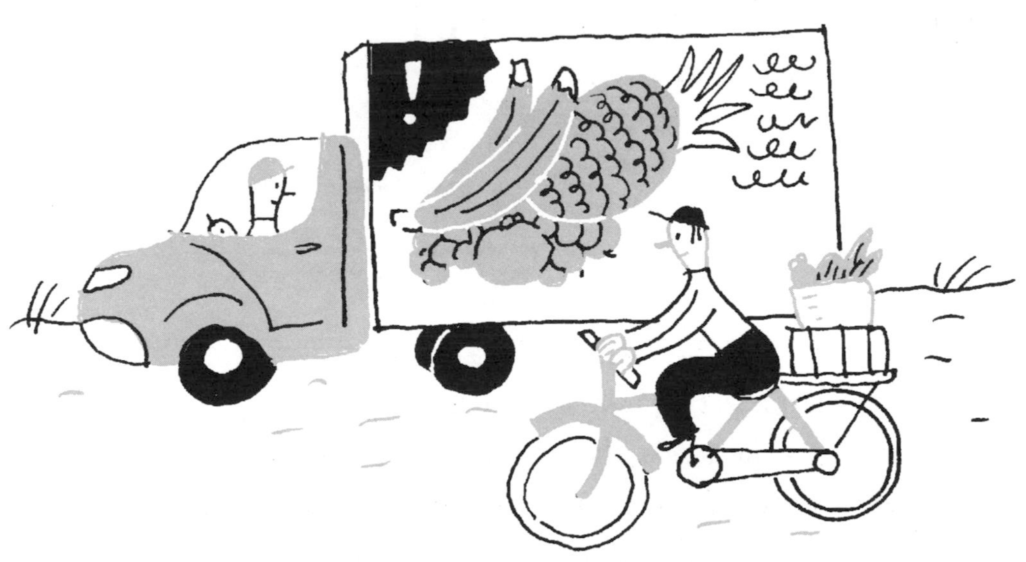

7 **To maintain biodiversity.** The multitude of seeds and breeds once enjoyed are disappearing fast. Eating (and saving seeds) from diverse plant cultivars and animal breeds from local farms, which are more likely to grow them, boosts biodiversity, an essential part of a healthy environment. Monoculture — raising vast quantities of only one cultivar or breed — spells devastation when disease strikes. In addition, monoculture takes the fun out of life. Imagine if only one kind of apple, the misnamed Delicious, were the only one left . . .

8 **To support our neighboring farms and farmers.** Eat local foods to ensure the health and longevity of our farm family businesses for today and tomorrow. Support farmers who bring us life's most seminal ingredient: our sustenance. Back farms that offer an alternative to current "standards" by providing safe, clean, and humane treatment of farm labor (and animals). Who wants to eat food brought to us through maltreatment?

9 **To preserve our culinary heritage.** Local food encourages traditions, whether they're as regionally distinctive as clambakes or as classic as Thanksgiving dinner. Strawberry picking in the spring, a visit to wine country, pumpkin harvest in the fall, and all the dishes traditionally accompanying the harvest bring us life and vitality, a shared experience of our world, a heritage we can savor and pass on to the next generation.

10 **To give us a just choice.** Eating local foods promotes a regionalized alternative to our food system, now consolidated into a handful of corporations that are not always looking after our interests. Local food supports a delicious, varied, just, and equitable food system.

I know it doesn't feel like it, especially if you're squeezed. But since the 1950s, the cost of food to consumers has made a steady decline. In 2008, food cost proportionately half of what it did in the '50s.

Local vs. Organic: Which Is Better?

Local is not necessarily organic. But which is better? From the perspective of this book: *Local organic and local sustainably produced food are best.*

Understanding the meaning behind this answer will help you make good decisions when you shop. Let's start with organic. Food labeled *organic* is required to be grown, raised, or produced using federally mandated rules. These standards outline allowable and forbidden materials and practices, which makes good sense. But they don't stress the integrated nature of farming, including the biological cycles necessary to healthy farming over the long haul. The organic label is also supported by strong agribusiness lobbies, which push for regulations to make their life easy (and our food not quite as safe).

Simultaneously, many of our local farmers are using safe, sustainable methods, which are the equivalent of or even better than established organic methods. They may or may not decide to become certified organic. If they opt out, it may be because their clients know and trust them, making certification unnecessary. Or perhaps they don't approve of its bias toward big agribusiness; they can't afford to follow the rules, which don't encourage small farms; they use another accredited system, such as Certified Naturally Grown; or they prefer to use their own, ecofriendly methods.

Buying certified organic food without thinking leaves out these farmers who grow delicious, safe food and also enrich their communities in numerous ways. Farmers are left behind, too, as stores and restaurants respond to our demand by stressing organic above local. It may support farming systems that are substantially better than conventional methods, but it also boosts the ballooning organic agribusiness and food often shipped from afar, using lots of fossil food as it ages. Yes, ages — organic does not mean fresh. Knowing a farmer and his or her values, or at least finding a trustworthy farm source, is the best way to procure foods raised in a manner that is healthier for you and for the earth, too.

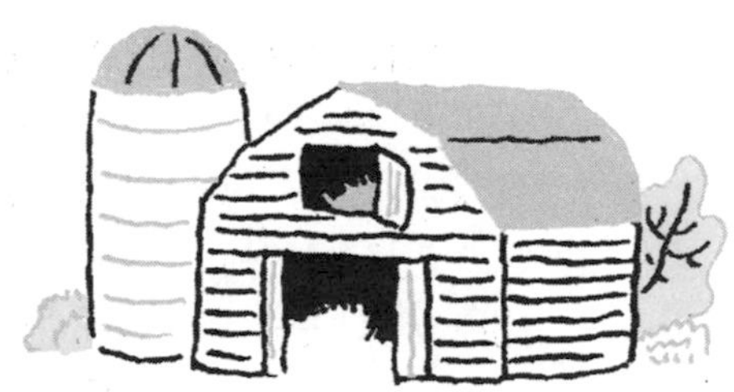

THE PRICE OF LOCAL FOOD

The farmers who produce the food that sustains us receive less on the dollar than ever before. Supporting your local food shed (system) puts more dollars in their pockets, helping to ensure their survival, but that doesn't save you money. The tips starting on page 15 help you meet your budget while boosting local farms and eating better, too. But first, let's talk about the price of local food.

COST VS. VALUE

The price of local food can equal or undercut food produced by conventional means and shipped to you from who-knows-where. But it can also be more. Rather than avoid the subject, or tell you to give up lattes in favor of farmers' markets (a favorite argument), I'll cut to the chase.

Every element of our current system supports a short-sighted emphasis on low-cost, high-volume production — no matter the quality or ultimate cost. To make matters worse, our food cost is artificially deflated because of huge corporate subsidies and is dependent on low-quality production, cheap labor, and ecologically unsuitable farming practices. How are small and medium farms to compete? Refocusing our food dollars on local sustainable farms may not always be cheap in the short term, but it's smart in the long term.

The bottom line? We're really talking about value, not price. We're comparing apples and oranges.

Are the following two carrots the same? The first is conventionally produced in dead soil, loaded with chemicals, and grown for endurance during its long trip to you, not for its flavor. The second carrot could be one of any number of cultivars, each distinctive, picked that day, produced by your farming neighbor (or at least regionally), grown in soil swimming with life, enhanced by sun and clean water, and harvested by workers treated in a humane manner. The story also applies to meat, dairy, and so on . . .

WHERE DID YOUR LAST MEAL COME FROM?

The story here is yours. Consider your last meal, or even the last snack you ate. Do you know where any of those ingredients came from? (And don't say "the supermarket.") Where were those foods grown, raised, or produced? Try to trace their origins.

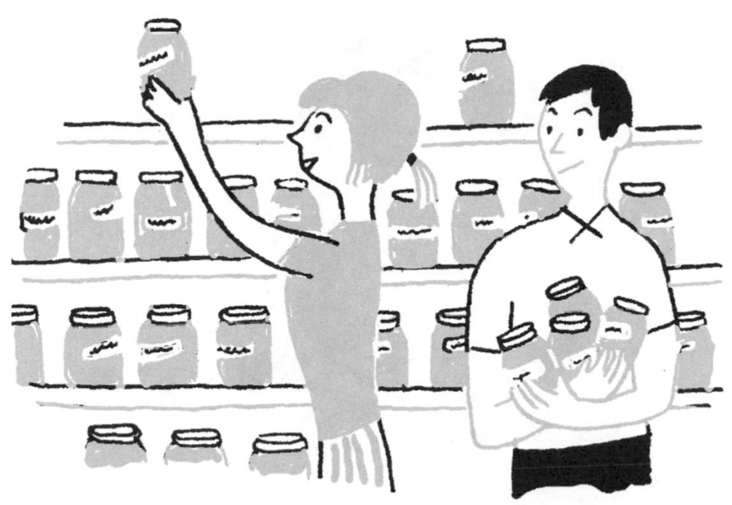

MONEY MATTERS

8 TIPS FOR CUTTING FOOD COSTS

1 **Become a smarter shopper.** Compare food prices. Never look at price alone, though. Also consider the quality and the edible quantity. Fresh food doesn't spoil as quickly as food that has already spent time in transit, so you'll end up with less waste. Stick with readily available staple items like carrots. Buy tasty green beans or Italian flat beans, not skinny posh French haricot verts. Skip the more expensive, prewashed meslcun mix and wash your own. Use the whole vegetable when you can — not just the beets, but their tops too. Buy in bulk when crops are plentiful; they're priced to move, especially at the end of the season.

2 **Join a CSA and pick your own.** CSA (community supported agriculture farm) membership and pick-your-own-farm visits are great values. Ask about incremental CSA payment plans, U-pick crops, and working memberships, where you barter labor for full or partial membership.

3 **Cook simply from scratch at home.** Food made from scratch is tastier and cheaper. (And don't fuss: local food almost cooks itself.) Pack healthful local foods for your own or your kids' lunches. Prepare extra dishes to eat during the week and freeze or preserve the surplus for later.

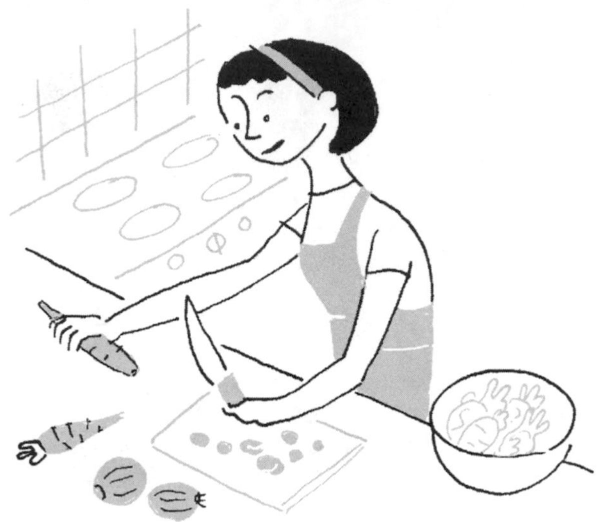

(8 Tips for Cutting Food Costs, *continued*)

4 **Dine out less or not at all.** Make local food an inexpensive "at-home" celebration. Invite friends for potluck suppers, where everyone brings a dish.

---

5 **Eat less meat.** Instead, experiment with alternative proteins like eggs and beans, which cost less to produce. For meat, join a buying club to cut costs.

---

6 **Locate low-income support programs.** For those who qualify, patronize venues that accept payment via Women, Infants, and Children (WIC); the Senior Farmers' Market Nutrition Program (FMNP); and the Supplemental Nutrition Assistance Program (SNAP, formally food stamps). More than half of farmers' markets now accept one or more of these payment options.

---

7 **Start a garden.** You can't eat closer to home than what's picked from your own backyard. If you don't have a yard, plant up a plot at a community garden. Other ways to do it yourself? Forage for wild foods with an expert or a club. Hunt or fish responsibly. If you're inexperienced, go with a neighbor or friend who is knowledgeable.

---

8 **Reprioritize your budget.** If you're able to, spend more on food and cut back on nonessentials.

Make the Most of the Seasons

Seasonal eating sits at the center of the locavore way. But, being contrary by nature, when I think of seasonal eating, I imagine quite the reverse. This is encapsulated in a postcard a friend sent me right after I moved to the country. It was divided into quarters, each with the same picture of a generic city street with a parked car. The photos were titled winter, spring, summer, and fall. I slapped the card on my fridge, so I see it every time I open the door. For me, the card typifies the way we've been taught to eat, in a manner divorced from nature, like a supermarket eggplant sitting in the four quarters of that postcard year-round.

Eating local food is different. We're able to catch the rhythms of nature, eating the best it has to offer, and extending its bounty throughout winter, the one dormant season for much of the United States. This requires an adjustment, which takes some practice but brings much joy. Here's how.

LEARN THE SEASONS BY SHOPPING FOR LOCAL FOODS

Once you've paid attention to what's in season around you by shopping locally, directly and indirectly from the farm, you'll have a solid sense of how to do it forever because seasons remain relatively constant (with all due respect to global warming weather variations, which can radically affect the normal flow of crops).

USE SEASONAL FOOD CHARTS

It's helpful to download the widely available seasonal produce charts, which will give you a good idea of what's available when. I especially like the Sustainable Table Web site (see Resources) because it has a link to each state with a clear, itemized chart. Download, then print it and put it on the fridge, in your car, or on the back of this book. For a sample seasonal flow, see page 33.

EAT SEASONAL FOODS UNTIL YOU'RE SATISFIED

I'm not a rigid locavore, but I never buy fresh corn or tomatoes in the winter. They're not worth it. One of the reasons I'm able go without strawberries, tomatoes, and other crops when they're out of season is that I savor them when they arrive until I'm sated.

So during the short strawberry season in late spring, my family and I try to eat berries until we can't. We eat plain strawberries out of hand, strawberries and cream, strawberry ice cream, strawberry shortcake, halved strawberries tossed with just a touch

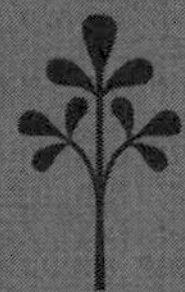

The Seasonal Eater

"There is a learning curve. You can't eat tomatoes at the beginning of the growing season, asparagus in October, or strawberries in August. But the reward is that you get to eat everything at its peak."

ELIZABETH KEEN

Indian Line Farm, Egremont, Massachusetts

"Our kitchen counters overflow with fresh produce in the summer. Food is lighter, often served raw or gently cooked. In wintertime, crates of potatoes, onions, and garlic keep cozy down in the basement. We bring out dried tomatoes, peppers, herbs and berries, frozen or canned foods; and we eat more soups, stews, and casseroles."

DAWN STORY

Local food activist, Virginia Grown, Charlottesville, Virginia of sugar and balsamic vinegar or kirsch (a cherry liquor), strawberry rhubarb crisp, sliced strawberries on yogurt — until our hands turn pink.

One year I wasn't on top of things and my daughter asked in a panic one day, "What about strawberries?" as if an alarm had gone off, programmed from years of waiting, then savoring. So, I drove down to the farm stand to pick up a basket of the season's last harvest. They were delightful, but we hadn't had our fill and so were disappointed; we knew we had to wait a year for the real taste of strawberries again.

Yes, a year. Seasonal eating means you're savoring food at its peak, knowing that it won't taste the same until next year. So I eat asparagus frequently in May and corn and tomatoes continuously and in every possible way in August. When I don't eat this way, like when I didn't get enough asparagus this season, the long dormant season is tougher and those Chilean asparagus — which are not remotely fresh and are probably sprayed with who-knows-what — begin to tempt me. Does that mean you should never ever eat anything out of season? That's your call. I have a long winter here in New England, but goals are always worth reaching for.

Wait, savor until you can't eat another bite, then wait and savor again.

GET CREATIVE WITH THE DORMANT SEASON

During the winter, when the soil is asleep, it's time to get friendly with all kinds of local foods — especially endless apples and pears, hearty vegetables such as winter squash and cabbage, and root vegetables like carrots, onions, and potatoes, along with local meat, poultry, maple syrup, eggs, and cheese. That's not all you'll eat, but try to make them the base of, or at least integrate them well into, your winter diet. For tons of ideas on what to do with winter (and all kinds of) foods see page 148, where they're listed by ingredient.

It helps to work the shoulder seasons, too — those in-between times. Depending on your climate, the first shoulder is late winter and early spring, when local crops from the harvest may have run out and new crops aren't ready to eat yet. This is a good time to start gardens, inside or out, and forage for early greens from the wild. The second shoulder season is around fall, again depending on where you live, but always just before your dormant season begins. It's a time for feasting on the last of the harvest and for foraging, as well. Prolong your garden's harvest by freezing or using traditional methods, such as canning, fermenting, or drying (see page 109).

STEP ONE

SHOP FOR LOCAL FOODS

The first step to becoming a locavore is to change how you shop. In the old days, you might have just plodded the aisles of your supermarket, pulling week-old lettuce from the produce bins and premade meals from the shelves. Everything you bought traveled thousands of miles to get to your shopping cart, losing its flavor each mile along the way.

As a local food shopper, you'll now load up on the best food you've ever tasted, and you'll enjoy finding it, too. Discover shockingly good flavors in heirloom vegetables, like zebra tomatoes from a roadside stand. Open a carton of mixed-color eggs, each with a bright orange, stand-up yolk. Savor the tangy taste of smooth, local goat cheese on a farm tour. Taste the extraordinary in the ordinary, like the potatoes and squash at your farmers' market. Or try the unfamiliar in your CSA farm share, like earthy celery root and hot habanero peppers. And notice truly fresh local milk, with the farm name on the front, right in your co-op or — surprise! — in your supermarket.

For the locavore, shopping becomes an integrated part of life, a treasure hunt, something to look forward to, with booty everyone can share. Sometimes it's a snap, like spotting apples in the supermarket with the farm's name right on the bag. Other times, it's laughably tough, like trying to find local beef when your apartment is 100 miles from the nearest cow. But it's an adventure that wakes up your senses and comes with a cadre of allies — from farmers to fellow shoppers — whose goal is to help you shop with the seasons to get the best food imaginable at its peak.

There are places to shop for locally grown and produced food everywhere. But it's no mistake that this section starts with direct-from-the-farm venues, like farmers' markets, then covers broader venues, like supermarkets. Buying food straight from the farm can't be beat, as you'll see, but retail shopping may also suit your lifestyle or locale. So most locavores do both.

Despite my favoritism, straight-from-the-farm venues are not one-stop shops — you're not likely to find toothpaste at the farmers' market. So, if you're used to buying everything at the supermarket, you'll have to organize your shopping a little differently. You might need to make separate trips, swinging by the farmers' market on your way back from work, stopping at a farm stand near a friend's house before a visit, or turning a trip to pick up your weekly CSA share into a family outing. For the amount of effort involved, the payoff is huge.

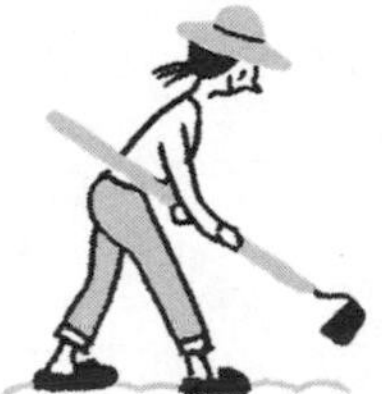

Farmers' Markets

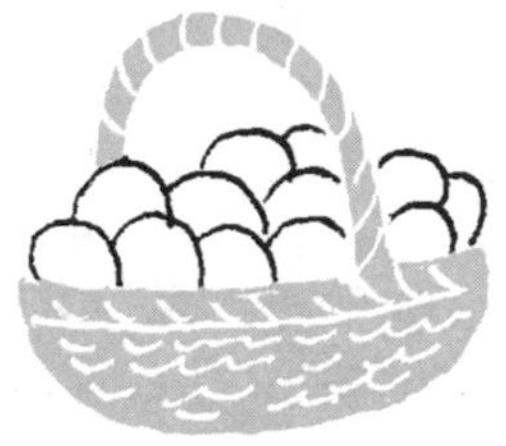

"The difference between a local field-ripened strawberry and a berry trucked in from distant states is enormous, and market shoppers figured that out really fast."

ELIZABETH RYAN

Market Farmer, Breezy Hill Orchard and Cider Mill, Staatsburg, New York

Why start our local food journey here? Visiting a local farmers' market, sometimes called a greenmarket, is the easiest way to instantly plunge into the world of fresh local food at peak flavor and connect face-to-face with the farmers who grow it.

Time to Shop?

One of the first things to learn about shopping at a farmers' market is simply when it's open. Unlike the supermarket, the hours of operation at a farmers' market vary: many open one day a week (sometimes for the whole day and sometimes just a few hours), while more active markets in large cities may be open as often as seven days a week. Peak market times are during the growing season, from a few months over the summer in Maine to year-round in Florida. (For the growing season in your region, follow the link to the Sustainable Table Web site in the Resources section and print out the crop availability chart for your state.)

It is also common for markets to remain open after the growing season ends, as well. These shoulder-month sales are likely to include greenhouse items, cold storage crops (such as apples and potatoes), value-added products (such as jams and pickles), nonperishable items, or less season-driven items like frozen butchered meats and aged farmstead cheeses.

MARKET TIME

GETTING READY FOR THE FARMERS' MARKET

- **Take cash.** Some farmers' markets don't take checks or credit cards.
- **Don't shop hungry.** Hungry people make irrational decisions without thinking clearly, grabbing what smells tasty or looks colorful.
- **Get an early start** when you can, as many markets run out of the best produce, especially at the beginning of the season.
- **Make a list, but be flexible.** If you take a shopping list, be prepared to adapt it to include unexpected finds.
- **BYO bags.** Take sturdy, reusable shopping bags. (The lifetime of one reusable bag replaces the one thousand plastic bags you'd need to carry the same quantity of food.) Or take a pretty basket or even a red wagon for your kids and then pile food all around them.

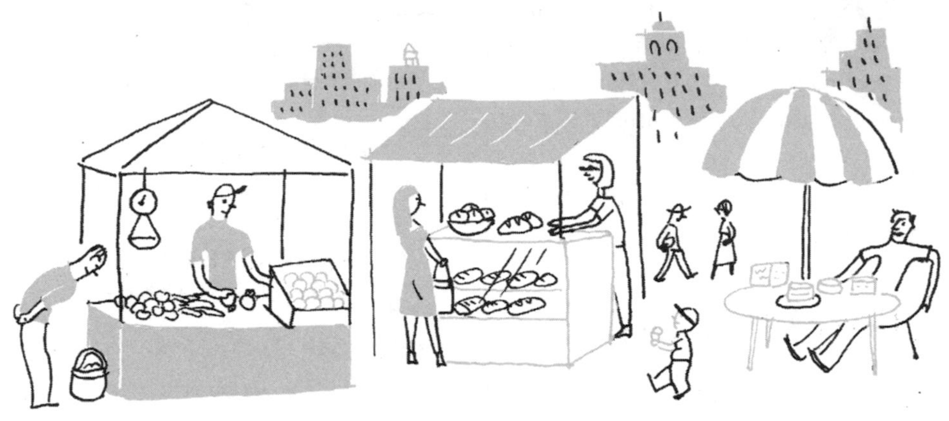

LOOK BEFORE YOU SHOP

Taking a quick tour of the market before you buy anything will serve you well. Check out the full spectrum of your food choices, learn the vendors' locations, and soak up the distinctive flavor of the market.

Let your eyes feast. Some vendors may even offer a taste of something they're particularly proud of, such as an heirloom apple or tomato. Be sure to look for and ask questions about ingredients you're not familiar with. Markets often offer cultivars (specific varieties) of fruits and vegetables, as well as meat and poultry breeds, that aren't available in supermarkets.

Learn each vendor's specialty. There may be a farmer who has a large selection of greens and can instruct you about which are bitter, sweet, crunchy, or tender. Or you can buy and try several varieties first, then go back the next week and purchase what strikes your fancy.

Look for hidden treasures. You'll find especially popular vendors with lines of hovering shoppers, but you're likely

Part of the pleasure of shopping at the farmers' market is the ephemeral nature of produce. And the mouthwatering wait until next season.

The Hardest Part

WAITING FOR THE GOOD STUFF

I hear repeatedly from farmers that seasonality is an especially difficult adjustment for new market shoppers. You can buy sweet peppers year-round in your supermarket, but at your farmers' market, you can buy them only when they're hanging on a plant not far from where you live. This timing takes a little getting used to, but you'll get the hang of the seasonal crop flow as you shop, and committed market shoppers soon become attached to the taste of produce at peak freshness. You'll learn to wait for the arrival of each fruit or vegetable and then eat it until it's gone. It will be worth the wait. Or if you like buying in bulk and storing and preserving foods, see pages 104–112.

to spot unexpected pleasures, too. Check out the less flamboyant vendors, stocked with regional meats in large ice chests, fresh eggs, local artisanal cheeses. Also look for value-added items, such as soups or sauces, breads, and other foods that are sometimes made from local ingredients.

Prioritize your purchases. Getting the big picture before you shop will allow you to plan on picking up the heaviest ingredients last. Meat, corn, potatoes, and cabbages can really weigh you down! A preshopping tour gives you a good sense of which fruits and vegetables are in peak season; there will likely be plenty of those. Over time, you'll see items come in and go out of season. Vendor tables that were overflowing with green beans at the beginning of bean season, for instance, will be reduced to a small crate by the tail end of it.

Every time I plunge in before I look around, I end up finding a perfect hard-to-find ingredient, such as *fraises du bois* — tiny alpine strawberries in season ever so briefly — after my bag is full and my budget has run out.

BE A SAVVY SHOPPER

Let your farmer be your teacher. Your best lessons come from the farmers' market and its community, so look around you, watch or ask farm vendors (and shoppers). These observations will teach you how to select and prepare foods. And of course, your farm vendors have been asked about storage and preparation tips a thousand times, so they know the answers!

Learn the food seasons. Take your cue from what's abundant. If it's in peak season, load up on it. Observe what comes in and out of season, overflowing and then dwindling. By the last market day, you'll understand basic crop flow for next year. Take notes or print out your own seasonal chart. Even I sometimes miss the short cherry season when I don't pay attention.

Learn new ways to cook. Keep an eye on the displays, which often teach you how to use specific foods. The maturity of a plant may also tell you how to prepare it: Small, young beet leaves sit in a bin next to other salad greens, signaling you to use them in a salad. Larger beet leaves may be bunched separately with other cooking greens, such as collards or kale, or sold still attached to the beets, signaling that they should be cooked. Written signs may also tell you how to prepare ingredients: cooking greens may be called "braising greens." So braise 'em. (See page 115 for more food preparation hints.)

Shop by category instead of by ingredient. Freshly harvested produce appears and disappears as it goes in and out of season. Ingredients you expected to arrive may have fallen prey to nature — a heavy rain finishing off the berries or deer eating the butternut squash crop. Make these uncertainties an asset by adopting a new shopping style. Rather than looking for specific ingredients, shop in general categories. Put "salad" on your list rather than specific salad ingredients. Shop for the best ingredients available rather than for specific kinds, selecting fruits or vegetables that are fine on their own or

STOCK UP FOR THE OFF SEASON

You may want to buy bulk produce in season and freeze or can it for the winter season. You may even get a deal if it's the end of the season, right before the frost, or if there's a bumper crop or slightly overripe or damaged produce. Deal or not, it's a great way to extend the season.

might also combine well. Shop for any grain, rice, or pasta, then pick out combinations of ingredients that could be thrown into any of these. You'll often find that nature makes sense; foods in season blend well together. Read recipes if you must, or just experiment!

Try something new. Certain foods get popular at the market and shoppers get into a rut, asking for Honey Crisp apples, Macouns, or whatever the current darling is, even after their time is past. Be willing to move on to what's next and might be better in its time. I know it's hard. I mourn the end of Macoun season, when the apples have lost the complexity of taste they had at the beginning of their run. But part of the pleasure of shopping at the farmers' market is the ephemeral nature of produce. And the mouthwatering wait until next season.

Some farmers sell their food right off their farm before and after the market season. Or they may have pick-your-own (often called U-pick) operations. If you're interested, just ask.

ALL AT ONCE

TIPS FOR SHOPPING FOR THE WEEK

- **Buy both perishable foods,** like raspberries, and produce that naturally holds well, such as carrots, onions, cabbage, and winter squash; slightly unripe ingredients; or value-added foods, such as cheese and maple syrup.
- **Simple rule: eat what's likely to go bad first.** Enjoy perishable items early in the week and move on to less-perishable ones later on.
- **Buy ample amounts of one or two staple items.** The easiest for me is mesclun mix (baby salad greens), which you can throw anything into and make a meal.
- **Prolong food's lifespan.** After you've finished the most perishable items, make a simple prepared dish that's a good keeper, such as soup or stew, a potato or grain casserole, or a hearty vegetable salad. (For tips on extending the season, see pages 104–112.)

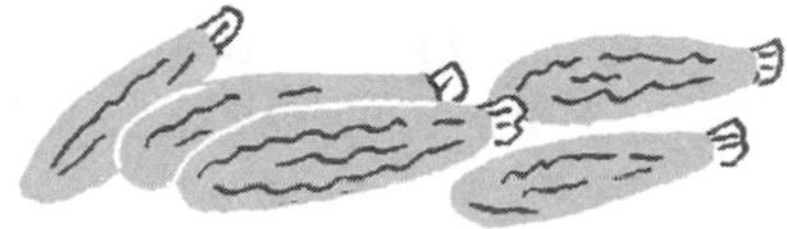

My First-Market-Day Ritual in Western Massachusetts

Here in the country, about the middle of May, we die-hard market fans, pale from the long winter months, make our way over to the Great Barrington Farmers' Market at the old train station. There are a few nods, smiles, and hugs, as we recognize each other and stop to chat. I head quickly over to the Stosiek family farm tent for a bag of mixed spring greens and arugula. Only 20 minutes later, at home or at my sister's house up on the hill, they're tossed in oil, salt, and a touch of vinegar. Boy, does that blow away the salads we've endured all winter long!

If You Buy It, They Will Come

Support your fledging farmers' market. Ideally, a market will have enough vendors for a range of ingredients, but markets have to start somewhere, and they grow only when community members patronize them. I've shopped in markets that started out with only four vendors, so I felt obliged to buy whatever was there. But they improved in size and quality as farm vendors and shoppers learned about each other's needs. Novice farmers came to understand that shoppers didn't want giant zucchinis, so they learned to harvest them earlier. Similarly, shoppers learned to cook with what was available for its freshness and flavor. Connections were made, and the markets grew.

Farmers' Markets Aren't Always Local

Strangely enough, it's possible to call something a farmers' market even when there are no farmers involved. Some are considerably more agricultural than others, and that means there will be more local foods on hand. Knowing the kind of market you're patronizing will help you find the food you're seeking.

A Level Playing Field

"A producer-only market creates a fair playing field for farmers because they don't compete against middlemen who may resell cheap goods from elsewhere. Of course many markets are not producer-only, and there are lots of gray areas where most markets operate, such as allowing tomato growers to bring in tomatoes from elsewhere when their season ends."

STACY MILLER

Executive Director, Farmers' Market Coalition

PRODUCER-ONLY MARKETS

"Producer-only" means that all of the market vendors grow or produce the products they sell; local food and farms are the market's focus. This description may seem like a given for a *farmers'* market, but it's not. Some local or regional farms may buy and bring in produce. Some vendors may not even sell food from regional farms at all, but procure their supply from a wholesale distributor, much like a supermarket.

Buying from producer-vendors gives you the advantage of connecting with the people who produce your food, so you can ask them questions about flavor, storage, shelf life, and cooking options, and what foods are coming in next.

Start by asking the market manager or one of the vendors if the market is a producer-only market. If it's not, ask which vendors are also producers. Then take veteran market farmer Elizabeth Ryan's advice: go directly to farm vendors and ask about what they're selling. Producer vendors will be deeply knowledgeable about how their food is grown, raised, or produced, and what to do with it. And of course, know your local crops' seasonality. You won't find local bananas in New England or mangos in Michigan any time at all.

Those interested in local food should encourage clear, specific point-of-origin labeling of produce and disclosure at markets that don't have a producer-only policy, so that shoppers know what they're buying and can make up their minds for themselves.

The Farmers' Market Boom

Although there are historical greenmarkets, such as Pike Place Market in Seattle, which started in 1907, the national market revival began in the 1970s and swelled from there. Between 1994 and 2008, U.S. markets more than doubled, for a total of 4,685. The USDA estimates that more than 30,000 farmers sell at farmers' markets, to at least 3 million community members annually, generating about $1 billion in purchases. The boom has increased demand to the point that most states are looking for more farm vendors.

BUY DIRECTLY FROM THE FARMER

In the industrial food system, only 20 cents out of every food dollar goes to farmers. The remaining 80 cents covers everything from packaging, transport, distribution, marketing, and slotting fees (paid to ensure product placement) to waste management.

A Tale of Two Markets

Here's a snapshot of two very different kinds of markets to give you a small taste of the endless market styles. Find local markets when you're traveling to get a sense of the distinctive quality of a region.

IN THE CITY: THE DALLAS FARMERS' MARKET

Texas is one of the few states that have a permanent market structure run by the city. Despite the name, farmers are just a component of the market, which encompasses 10 acres of wholesale, retail, and produce markets smack in downtown Dallas. Built in 1941 and open 362 days a year, local produce generally starts in April with strawberries and continues through the end of October. Sales from the 55 farm vendors are mostly in seasonal produce, but farmers also bring items like eggs and meat from a Texas meat consortium of several ranches that raise their cows on pasture rather than on grain. (See page 75 for more about grass-fed meat.)

The market is not a producer-only market, although many vendors sell their own crops. Recently, market administrator Janel Leatherman started to work toward clearly delineating what food was locally produced, using better signage and vendor placement. Farm checks have just been initiated to confirm that supplier farms sell only what they grow, although farm vendors are still permitted to buy-in supplies if they work the market 7 days a week.

The market's mission is to provide its customers with healthful, fresh,

GETTING YOUR HANDS ON THE FOOD

At some markets, kids — and adults still full of wonder — get a solid sense of their food and its origins through touch and talk. At the Virginia Beach market, there's a simulated cow that kids can milk. This may not measure up to the real thing, but kids unlikely to visit a farm still learn that milk doesn't come from jugs and cartons. At the same market, farmer Elsie Creekmore, now 87, has been coming for 30-plus years with her popular butterbeans, which she shells by the thousands. She's often helped by family and market shoppers, some of whom come back every year to pitch in. Do the beans taste better when you shell them yourself?

and affordable locally grown food and to help better the community. The city just renovated two buildings: one for a restaurant and specialty food store and the second for a Texas wine store, a new resource for locally produced wine. From her office, Leatherman can see the Dallas skyline and the market, ringed with other wholesalers and new townhouses.

IN A TOWN: THE MORGANTOWN FARMERS' MARKET

There are many entrance points to the open-air Morgantown Farmers' market, located 70 miles west of Pittsburgh in Morgantown, West Virginia. It started in 2001 in a donated city parking lot, nestled between a private building and an old church. This producer-only market, filled with farmers' pop-up tents, started on Saturday afternoons with about seven farmers selling vegetables, meat, and eggs.

Today the 27 vendors, selling a wide range of ingredients and value-added products, have turned the market into a one-stop shop. A local beef co-op sells grass-fed meat. Several egg vendors help meet the huge demand, but they always sell out. Heirloom apples, greens, and tree fruit, including pawpaw (an indigenous American fruit described by locals as a kind of culinary cross between a banana and a mango with papaya-like seeds), are particularly popular. A shiitake grower sells mushrooms cultivated on logs in the woods, a form of agriforestry that's increasing in popularity. Baked goods, such as pies, are a hit. A caterer makes homemade pierogies using local potatoes.

The market has been tracking its gross sales during the 23-week season, which have grown from $110,00 to $175,000 in the last year. "No doubt, the market has become a social hub," says Stacy Miller, who worked as market manager when she was a student and is now executive director of the Farmers' Market Coalition. "It takes only 15 minutes to buy produce, but folks are there standing around with dogs and chatting for 2 hours," she says. "Even local college students are starting to get themselves up on Saturdays after partying the night before so they can shop the market."

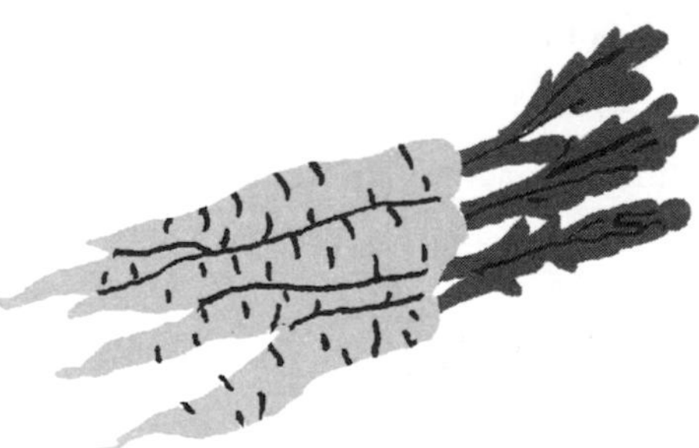

THE SEASONAL MARKET

While your region may have different seasons, this list will give you a good idea of how local food varies over a season. Note that it is not an inclusive list, just a sampling, and the length of availability for any item of produce varies. For example, lettuce may start in early spring and continue until it gets cold, while cherries have a very short season. And some foods have several seasons. But don't worry too much about details. Start here, then download your regional chart from Sustainable Table (see Resources).

- **Late winter:** maple syrup (but holds through the seasons)
- **Spring:** asparagus, spinach, strawberries, peas, sugar snaps, cherries, young greens, chives, and more
- **Summer:** carrots, green beans, summer squash, zucchini, corn, tomatoes, cucumbers, peppers, eggplant, lettuce, potatoes, tomatoes, blueberries, and much more
- **Later summer:** melons, cabbage, peaches, and grapes
- **Fall:** apples, winter squash (including pumpkins), sweet potatoes, and more
- **Year-round:** dairy (eggs, milk, cheese), often available most of the year; meat, often slaughtered when the grass is finished but available frozen year-round; fish, depending upon location

The Market Farmer, Heartbeat of the Farmers' Market

ELIZABETH RYAN, FARMER

Breezy Hill Orchard and Cider Mill, Staatsburg, New York

Knoll Crest Egg Farm, Clinton Corners, New York

Stone Ridge Orchard, Stone Ridge, New York

Elizabeth Ryan, a pretty woman in her early 50s with long gray-blonde hair, is one of the many growers selling goods at farmers' markets across the country. Her operation is a large one by East Coast standards, with 251 acres in fruit trees and berries at Breezy Hill Orchard and Cider Mill, and 16,000 free-range chickens at Knoll Crest Egg Farm. She's also recently acquired Stone Ridge Orchard, which has a popular U-pick operation. At the peak of the season, she sells to 15 markets in the region, some as close as the next town and some as far away as Queens, New York, 100 miles to the south.

A HISTORY IN FARMING

"Willa Cather's *My Antonia* is my story," says Elizabeth Ryan. Her great-grandfather broke sod in the Iowa wilderness in 1875.

Her grandparents were "populist rebels" who resisted change, and she's followed in their footsteps. Even by 1970, when her grandfather died, they were still feeding more than 20 people a day (both family and farm workers), raising their own chickens, grinding wheat for bread, and preparing most everything from scratch.

Fresh out of Cornell University, Elizabeth and her then-husband Peter Zimmerman bought their first farm, Breezy Hill Orchard, in 1984.

Luckily, the farm's retired owners were looking to mentor the young farmers who bought their land. Procuring a mortgage was tough then, and hasn't gotten much easier for Hudson Valley farmers. Just three years ago the bank told Elizabeth that the region could support only boutique farms with second incomes!

FARMING PRACTICES: THE CHOICES WE MAKE

Breezy Hill Orchard and Stone Ridge grow tree fruits — apples, pears, peaches, plums, cherries, nectarines — as well as strawberries, raspberries, and blackberries. In the damp Northeast, it's difficult to grow organically, but Elizabeth uses as few synthetic products as possible, searching out those with the lowest residuals, and using integrated pest management (IPM; see page 223), like dispensing ladybugs and little beetles to eat the mites that can damage her crop.

"I remember the first time I saw a young mom put our cider in her baby's bottle. 'This is the only juice I give my kids,' she told me. That's such a huge responsibility," Elizabeth says.

The law in most states insists that farmers kill bacteria in cider, but Elizabeth doesn't pasteurize because it "kills the soul of cider," turning it into highbrow apple juice. Instead, her cider is passed over UV light, which kills the bacteria while preserving its flavor.

Every market day, people ask why Elizabeth's egg farm isn't organic, and it's a good question. The laying hens are free range; no hormones or antibiotics are used. Their eggs are sustainable but aren't organic, because Elizabeth often can't find enough organic feed to keep her large farm running. And, when available, organic feed costs two and a half times more than standard grain, which Elizabeth feels would result in a selling price steeper than her customers would tolerate. In fact, the overall cost of farming is so high that costs for feed and fuel put her in debt last year.

FARM WORKERS

A solid proportion of the farm's labor force is made up of immigrants. "They have the reverence and skill set for farming," says Elizabeth, "and I make an effort to run a family-oriented business. The farm is like a village or tribe, one for all and all for one. I want to give immigrants the best life they can have here."

Breezy Hill's nonimmigrant workers, usually twenty-somethings from affluent families, often have trouble adjusting to the farming life, which includes hard work all the time and noncompartmentalized jobs where everyone "does what needs to be done until it's done."

THE WEATHER AND OTHER DISASTERS

No matter how stable the farm, a farmer's living rises and falls with the weather.

"We're still subject to epic forces of nature, hurricanes, frost, and hail," Elizabeth says. "When the region's fruit crop was wiped out three

THE FORCES OF NATURE ARE PART OF WHAT YOU EAT

Even with tiny dings from the spring hailstorm, those Honey Crisp apples taste sweet and juicy. It's been cold, but you can wait another week for those berries to come in. Or perhaps the constant rain destroyed the crop. Forces of nature are going to affect any farm-fresh food you buy, so consider it part of what it means to buy local foods. It can be frustrating, but it gives you a window into the forces of nature. So, go with the flow if the crop comes early, late, or occasionally not at all — or if it looks funky but tastes great. Remember that you reap the benefits of weather, too, when an abundance of sweet tomatoes comes in because of an ideal growing season.

years ago, it was a wake-up call to me as a grower — there are things that you cannot fix or will away."

A few years ago, Breezy Hill had a catastrophic fire of what Elizabeth calls "biblical proportions." Despite the 150 firefighters at work, the destruction of buildings, equipment, and land was devastating. The outpouring of affection for Breezy Hill included a benefit dinner, arranged by famous chefs and food writers in Manhattan, where Elizabeth was a founding member of the Union Square Market.

A year later, Elizabeth chaperoned one of the employees to court after he ran a stop sign. The judge recognized her and told the court that he'd been at the fire. Then he waved her and her employee home, telling the court how he loved the farm and hoped it would stay afloat.

THE MARKET VENDOR

During the market season, Elizabeth's farms revolve around the markets they supply. She is already concerned with what the weather will be like two or three days before market opens. How will she juggle her supply with the demand that is up on good weather weekends? Do they make 100 apple pies, or 10 because it'll be raining and no one will show?

Days vary, but on Saturdays the farm does four to six markets at a time — one in her home town, a few close by, and one as far away as Long Island City. She spends a chunk of her time "looping the loop," visiting those markets, hanging out with customers, and troubleshooting. This year some of the trucks that service the Manhattan market will stay in town to save on fuel.

Traffic is a problem; by the time they arrive at city markets, they need to unload fast, essentially setting up an outside store in two to three hours before the customers arrive. This timetable means pulling out tables, setting up scales, hanging banners, and setting out as many as 50 signs to label everything, as well as assembling heavy tents that are tricky to set up.

Elizabeth likes intimate markets or slower weekday markets where she can get to know the families and their names. About a third of her customers are regulars, and that percentage is even higher at locations outside of the city.

Value-added products, like cookies and pies, are a big boon to market farmers. Breezy Hill turns fruit into chutneys and popular pies. And with people a generation or two away from pie making, Elizabeth often finds herself giving advice to those who want to bake their own.

Despite the hard work, Elizabeth adores market days. "A lot of what we get out of the farmers' market is the love," she says.

SOCIAL JUSTICE AND LOCAL FOOD

When you buy from farms that treat their workers fairly, you are helping to limit the cruel conditions for farm workers. And although it's not always possible to find out, knowing your farm vendor or visiting his or her farm (or Web site) may give you some idea of how the staff is treated. Your food dollar votes for everything it takes to make that food, including the treatment of the people who grow it.

Farm Stands and U-Pick Farms

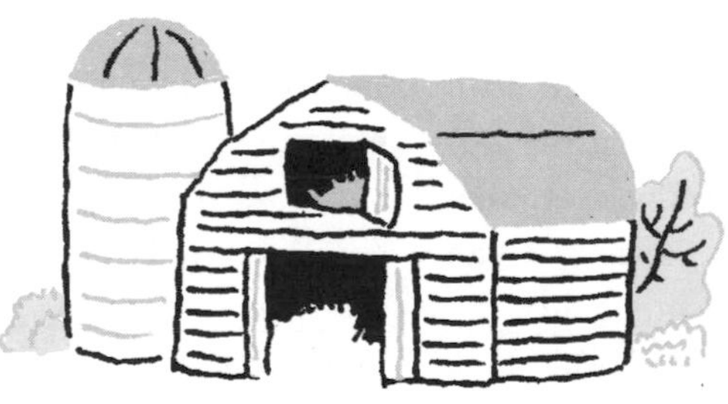

"There are four things people will always pull over for — strawberries, apples, corn, and tomatoes."

RAY McENROE

McEnroe Organic Farm, Millerton, New York

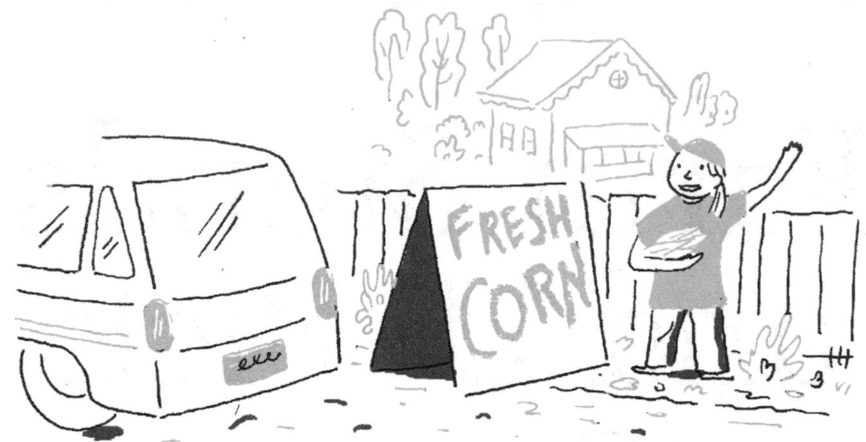

Roadside farm stands vary widely in size, style, and formality, giving them lots of local character. On the small end of the scale, my neighbor on Pixley Hill sets out her raspberries in plastic cups in a cooler with a handwritten sign marked "$1." The stand, if you can even call it that, is unmanned; just slip your money into a box. Locals look for her sign during the brief raspberry season. Blink and you miss it. On the other end of the spectrum sits McEnroe's Organic Farm Stand in Millerton, New York, a 700-acre organic farm with a large farm store out front selling everything from vegetables, grain, and poultry to fresh-baked apple pies. Between these two extremes, thousands of markets stocked with just-picked fruits and vegetables, humanely raised meat, and value-added products await your business.

Anything you can purchase at a farmers' market can also be bought at a farm stand, and so there are similar guidelines for shopping. But farm stands are open more hours, giving you more flexibility to fit in your shopping. Often, farm stands also provide fewer choices simply because one farm (or maybe a handful) is producing for it. Freshness at farm stands can be hit or miss — although the food is often harvested that day, as it would be for a farmers' market, it can sit out for much longer than if it were at the market. Just as at any store, freshness depends on how swiftly items sell.

Just like farmers' markets, there's no one style for farm stands. But unlike a market, which has general rules, a stand is an independent business where the boss (the farmer) sets the standards.

Get the Best from Your Farm Stand

Farm stands are often just what you expect them to be: farmers selling their own crops in a small store in front of their farm. But some of them also include food from other local farmers to fill in what they don't grow. Others buy from distributors to supplement their crops. And some aren't farm stands at all — just stores tricked up with farm charm. It's not difficult to tell what you're buying if you stop and think.

How can you tell? Look for box labels or signs that say "Our own blueberries are in right now." Ask, "What's grown here?" Like everyone else, farmers like to talk about their work. Is it their farm? "What's coming in especially good this season?" You may get an answer like this one: "The corn came in late because of the weather, but the kernels are full and sweet now." Or the farmers may recognize you as someone especially interested and add: "I used to grow only the super-sweet corn because it holds well and people love the sugary flavor, but I'm also growing an heirloom variety that has an old-fashioned corn flavor." Sometimes they'll even steer you

Pick It Yourself

U-pick farms dot the countryside, and are often a component of farm stand businesses. Visiting them is about as close as you can get to a locavore's dream come true. Here the food is where it belongs: on the farm, surrounded by nature, accompanied by the farmers who grew it, with fellow food-lovers picking it.

What could be a better way to explain to your kids where their food comes from than to have them pick it themselves? Turn the annual harvest of crops into a family ritual that includes low-cut trees laden with orchard apples; cherries, white to hot pink to burgundy, hanging like polka dots against the sky; or ripe strawberries in neat rows perfuming the mountain air.

Just follow the farmer's directions when picking. They know what's best and where to pick it. Respect their instructions and their farm, and enjoy these memorable adventures. (To find a U-pick farm near you, follow the Web link for Pick Your Own in Resources.)

to something good that doesn't look quite right. "These tomatoes don't look great, but that's because their variety is shaped that way. I had one in a salad for lunch and it was fabulous."

If you're still in serious doubt about the origins of the food at a farm stand, check out what's seasonal. Bananas are always one of those great markers. A farm stand that sells bananas may still sell their own stuff, but it means they're selling other items from outside the region (or country) as well. Again: ask.

Farm Stand and U-Pick Farms Near You

Far more farm stands exist than any other direct buying source, and there's no one way to find them, especially as the USDA does not, as of yet, track them. But here are some ways to look, and looking is part of the local food adventure.

As with all local detective work, ask your friends, particularly those interested in food. Try farmers' markets; someone may be a vendor at an inconvenient market but have a farm stand that's close to you. Check with local nonprofits that support agriculture, as well as cooperative extension agents in your region (see Resources). Many areas publish farm stand maps. Try the chamber of commerce or your local agriculture advocacy group. If you don't know who they are, try your town government or a kindred nonprofit, such as an environmental group or land conservancy. Ask at the local food co-op; the produce manager or someone shopping in produce might know, or you may find signs at the co-op that list names. Look 'em up or Google 'em. Keep your eyes peeled. I've found unexpected treasures while I'm just driving around, and sometimes I even forget them until I drive by them again. Look on local calendars for food-based events, farm tours, harvest-based celebrations, especially, but not exclusively, those at farms. And, of course, look at the many Web sites starting on page 227.

Wineries

America is one of the great wine-producing countries. Many wineries have wine bars, tasting rooms, and restaurants that are open to the public. Wine trails will take you from vineyard to vineyard, a terrific way to vacation. I'm still moved by the image of orange poppies growing between rows of grapevines on the Bonterra vineyard in Mendocino County, California. (For more about local wine, see page 166.)

Goodness Grows

AL PETERSON

Peterson Produce, Delano, Minnesota

Peterson's Produce is located on Route 12, 35 miles east of Minneapolis, outside the suburban belt and a stone's throw from the small town of Delano. It's a cedar shake stand with a corncob painted on its side, along with their motto, "Goodness Grows." The 25-year-old business is popular for its busy location, fresh crop, good service, and pretty presentation. "When the flowers come in," Al Peterson says, "my wife Jean puts up a wall of flowers. It really brings them in. She redecorates every week."

Al, now 60, married into Jean's family farm after his business lagged and Jean was laid off from her job. They teamed up with her brother to convert the 140-acre farm into a produce business with 55 acres (now down to 20 acres) of vegetables. They tried selling their produce at farmers' markets, by wholesaling, and by operating a second stand, but the one farm-located stand stuck.

"My wife and I have kind of a role reversal," he says. "She's less social and enjoys the physical work out on the farm. I have a bad back and prefer working directly with customers, chatting and having fun with people."

Typical customers are locals and suburbanites who regularly travel to the farm. The stand is open seven days a week from 8 AM to 7 PM, but it's not unusual to see headlights out front at 10 PM from customers stopping by to buy produce using the honor system. (One such customer moved to Delano 15 years ago after seeing the stand's moneybox full, unlocked, and unmanned.)

The Petersons start planting in April and finish up at the end of September with the killing frost. Pumpkins are their most popular crop, covering 10 acres and bringing out families to pick their own every year, including parents who picked when they were young and who now bring their kids in tow. They've pared down their remaining crops to those they can physically manage, including green beans, garlic, and tomatoes, buying the rest at neighboring farms. (They sell 50 to 200 dozen ears of corn a day.) But early on, they made the decision not to buy-in from farms far afield, a hard call considering how ravenous their clients are for farm-fresh foods.

"They'd be happy to buy Georgia peaches. But keeping it local maintains our identity," Al says. "Farmers do everything, from petting zoos to making pies from their apples. We're a farm stand selling local farm foods. That's what we do best."

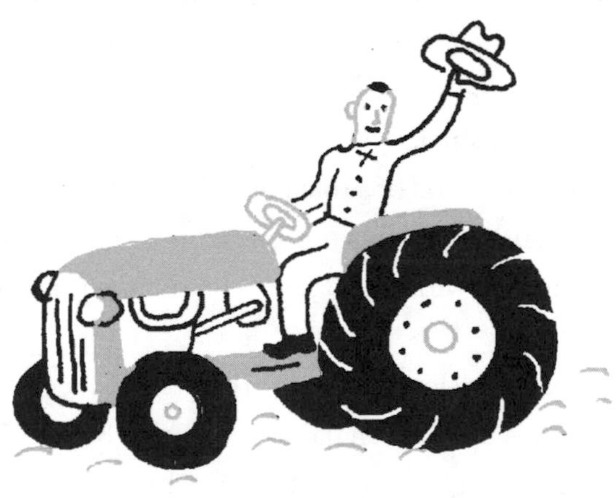

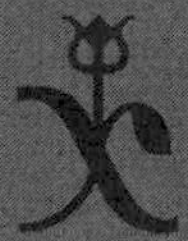

What It Means to Be Sustainable

"Sustainable farming is a process; it can't be attained. You're always trying to do things better, but you are never there, always just getting there. If you sign on, you make the commitment to do things in an environmentally friendly way. We went from thousands to $18 a year in chemicals, but we aren't certified organic. For me, sustainable means that it has to be profitable for the farm and good for the community, as well as providing jobs and good food for the community."

AL PETERSON
Peterson Produce, Delano, Minnesota

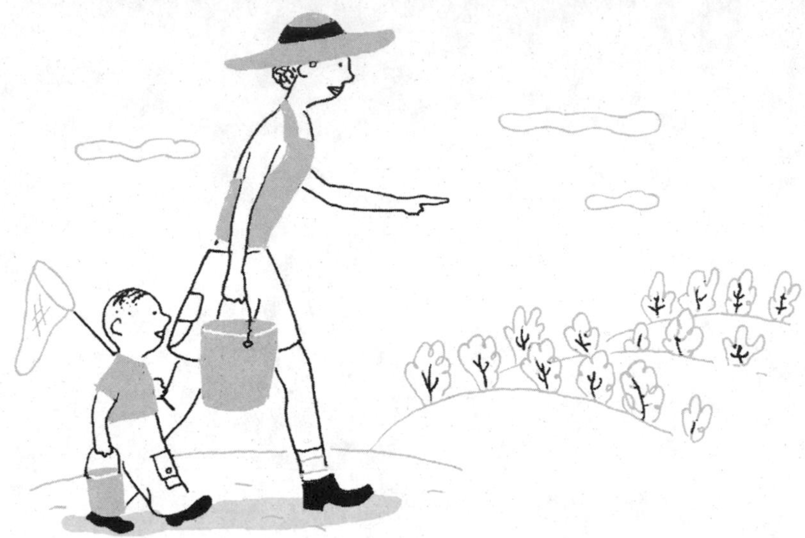

Ready to Pick Your Own?

Listen to your farmers; they know the ropes.

Respect their land; don't trample crops or alarm farm animals.

Pick what's ripe unless directed otherwise.

Wear sunblock and a hat if it's sunny.

Cover your arms and legs when picking prickly crops like raspberries.

Take your own baskets or bowls, one for each picker.

Eat before you go or you'll go wild.

Enjoy!

Rules of on-farm sales vary from state to state, but most allow roadside farm stands.

Community Supported Agriculture

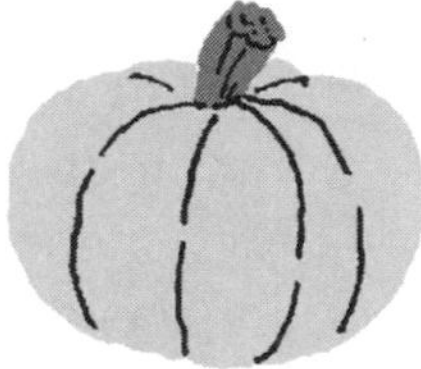

"I knew that there had to be a way — something cooperative, people combining their abilities, expertise, and resources — to bring the people producing the food in touch with the people eating it."

ROBYN VAN EN

Indian Line Farm, Egremont, Massachusetts
Cofounder of the CSA movement in the United States

Grab a bag of this morning's harvest, brimming with summer vegetables, on your way home from work. Pick tiny pear-shaped tomatoes right off the vine with your kids. Chat with your farmer about whether to choose the carrots, baby bok choy, or odd-looking kohlrabi.

Join a CSA (community supported agriculture) farm and bring home a weekly share of the harvest over the growing season and often beyond it. CSAs are located everywhere — in the city, country, and suburbs — with pickups on the farm and sometimes in your own neighborhood. They offer a unique window into fresh, sustainably raised, local food, as well as a chance to directly support your local farm and farmer.

Joining is a personal way of answering the question, "Where does my food come from?" Members share the risk and the bounty, connect with the farm and the farmer, and witness the flavorful flow of nature as crops go in and out of season. But unlike shopping at the farmers' market or farm stand, where you dip in and out as you need, membership requires a financial commitment and may hold you to specific harvest and pick-up days.

Thousands of families feel that the rewards of membership are worth the effort. Find out in this chapter if joining a CSA is a good local food route for you.

What Is a CSA?

"CSA" stands for *community supported agriculture*. Although it denotes a kind of farming, the term has also come to mean the farm itself. CSA members, sometimes called shareholders, agree to support an environmentally responsible farm and farmer by paying up-front costs before the growing season

Join a CSA and get a grocery bag or so of sustainably raised farm-fresh food on a regular basis. Pick-up days are especially satisfying if you can visit the farm, but even city slickers look forward to their weekly bag of startlingly fresh produce, and many visit the farm at least once a season.

VISIT YOUR CSA

Most CSAs have at least one event each season to bring their members together to enjoy the farm. Even if you live far from your CSA, you should consider attending. Or you can plan an outing on a day when you can pick something yourself, such as raspberries or sugar snaps. My first membership culminated in a harvest party where, on a blustery fall day, members and their children, including my daughter, chose pumpkins from the field to take home for Halloween.

and sharing in both the bounty and the risk of the harvest. While all CSAs operate in their own way, these principles remain constant.

What does that mean in practical terms? Generally, CSA members pay for their seasonal harvest up-front, help to finance the farmer's costs, and then pick up their share of produce during the course of the season. Members receive food harvested the morning they pick it up or sometimes the day after (especially in the city). Those living close to the farm (or close enough for a visit) get to meet their farmer and see how their food is grown and, if they like, harvest some of it, too.

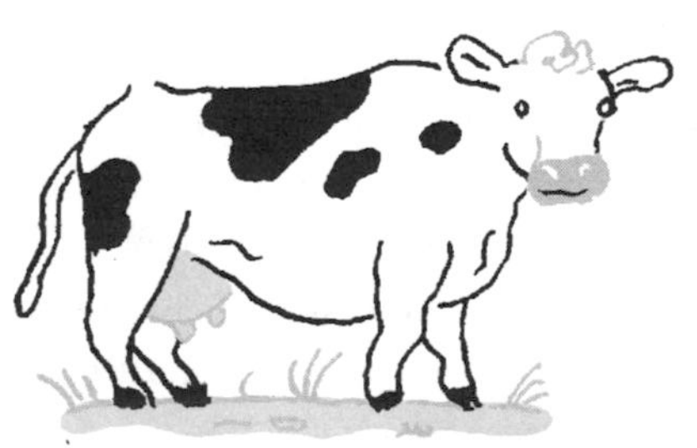

How often do you pick up your share? Harvest day is usually once a week, often with a choice of two pick-up days. Farmers try to accommodate their members by selecting times that are convenient for working people.

Where do you pick up? If you live near the farm, you might pick it up directly on harvest day. If you live in the city or suburbs, you should be able to find a CSA that drops off shares at a pick-up location near you.

What do you get? CSAs tend to focus on produce, with a strong emphasis on vegetables, but they may include other ingredients with membership or as a la carte items for an extra fee. Commonly these include milk, eggs, cheese, meat or poultry, fruit, and breads or baked goods that are prepared at the farm or brought in by other farmers or artisan bakers. Some CSAs also grow pick-your-own crops — generally fruits and vegetables that are very plentiful and/or require a lot of labor to harvest. (This opportunity makes for a great family outing.) These crops may include peas, beans, berries, cherry tomatoes, flowers, herbs, and more.

On pick-up days, produce is separated into bins for easy access. You'll know exactly how much to take because a menu board or individual signs will instruct you. Often, members are invited to take a certain amount (say, eight tomatoes) or to weigh out produce (half a pound of lettuce). Many CSA farmers, however, try to make it easier by not burdening their members with too much weighing. Some CSAs offer a choice between two vegetables, or you can select, say, five of seven items. That way, if you hate turnips, you may be able to choose beets or carrots instead. You may also receive unusual varieties of familiar foods because they are raised for flavor, not durability. (See Heirloom Produce, page 192.)

Share sizes differ, but most CSAs offer at least two sizes — a larger share for a family and a smaller share for one-to-two-person households. When crops are plentiful, shares may be large. On average, members receive an ample bag of produce per week. Your fresh share is raised using ecofriendly methods.

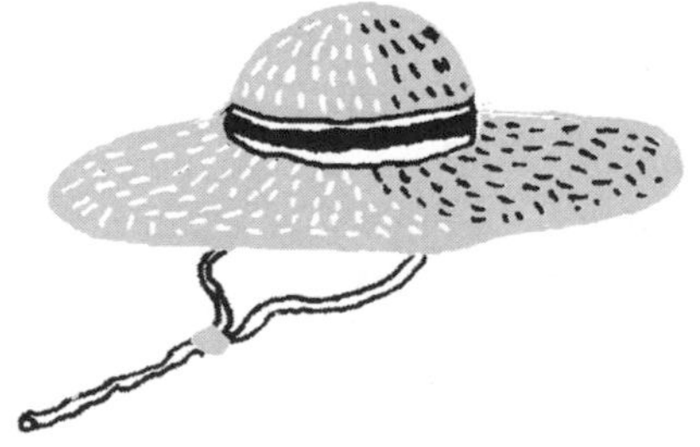

How long does a share last? Generally CSA shares run for the course of the growing season or a little beyond; some go as long as 42 weeks or offer a separate winter share of greenhouse and root vegetables. The length of the shares will depend on both the weather of your region and the style of your CSA.

What does it cost? The cost of a share varies according to the length of the season and the size of your share. According to an independent study, an average CSA share costs less than half of what you would pay for the same amount of organic produce in a supermarket. Also, for those who pick up at the farm or who may want to make a special excursion, a CSA's pick-your-own crop features can be a tremendous savings, especially at season's end when they may even be unlimited!

What if you're on a tight budget? Some CSAs encourage working memberships that barter farm work for full or partial membership. (This option can be enormous fun, in addition to saving you money.) Many CSAs will

CSAs Firsthand

"Often my CSA members have no idea what veggies look like when still attached to the plant, and I see folks having 'ah-ha' moments frequently here."

ELIZABETH KEEN, FARMER

Indian Line Farm CSA, Egremont, Massachusetts

"I bring my grandchildren to pick beans and tomatoes with me, to watch things grow, and to harvest them firsthand."

MARION STEIN, MEMBER

Indian Line Farm CSA, Egremont, Massachusetts

"We are competitive with supermarkets, but this isn't just about money savings and it's not about convenience. It's more convenient to pick what you want from a grocery store. This is not one-stop shopping. But you can feed lots of mouths from a CSA membership if you have the resourcefulness, curiosity, and flexibility to do it."

ROB WOOD

Spoutwood Farm, Glen Rock, Pennsylvania

let customers pay in installments or by a sliding scale, to encourage low-income families to join. Some offer an opportunity for community members to donate CSA shares, which then go to local food pantries.

Is CSA Membership Right for You?

Becoming a CSA member may be an exhilarating experience, but it's not for everyone, so review this list before taking the plunge.

Does it fit into your schedule? Think about what honestly works for you before you sign up. Although Indian Line Farm in Egremont, Massachusetts, has grown to its projected membership size, they still lose 10 percent of their members each year, mostly because the location, day of the week, or pick-up times are inconvenient.

Do you cook? If you don't like to cook at all, you can still integrate farm-fresh foods into your diet with ingredients like local milk, cheese, fruit, and pre-washed greens. But CSA membership requires you to pick up some foods that will need preparation. You don't have to cook complex recipes, because really fresh produce is so shockingly tasty that often the less you do, the better; some cooking will still be required though.

Can you be flexible with what's in your share? CSA members have to focus their meals around what they get each week. Strict pre-pick-up planning is out, although many things are available week-to-week and you may have a heads-up on what's coming next. But you can't be a control freak. Don't plan on cooking a butternut squash soup

FEEDING THE HUNGRY

The large-scale Food Bank Farm in Hadley, Massachusetts, was the first CSA with the primary mission of helping to feed the hungry. It gives half of its annual harvest to those in need, averaging 200,000 pounds of fresh produce each year. Not far from there, in Berkshire County, my home turf, I helped boost the much smaller Share the Bounty program, which asks for community donations for CSA shares to be delivered to local food pantries. This low infrastructure system can accommodate donations of any size, which are then consolidated to buy pantry shares each season. It's an easy thing to start up on your own.

The original Japanese CSA-style farms, with their farm-to-member arrangement, are called *teikei* in Japanese, or "putting the farmer's face on food."

if you aren't sure it's come in yet, but feel free to plan to make a vegetable soup with whatever's been picked that day. The best plan of action is to make your meal plans once you've picked up your share.

Are you willing to try new foods? The majority of your share is user-friendly produce, food you're likely to be familiar with, such as lettuces, tomatoes, and corn. But a share may introduce you to new ingredients you haven't cooked (or even seen) before, from braising greens to kohlrabi. Many CSAs give out recipes, other members may offer tips, and, if all else fails, recipes are plentiful online and in cookbooks. If cooking new foods doesn't interest you, a CSA share may not be for you. But if you're excited to try something new, give membership a try.

Are you excited to visit the farm? Although it may be hard to say before you begin, you probably have a general idea of whether visiting a farm, harvesting some of your own food, or picking your own flowers seems like an adventure or a chore. Members who visit the farm generally find that the connection they make picking their food at its source is as valuable as the food itself.

Can you deal with the bounty? CSA shares vary, but when they are ample, some members feel overwhelmed. While it's silly to take what you won't use, members may feel obligated to do so because they've already paid for it. (You don't have to!) But if you do, it helps to be able to prolong the life of some of the bountiful crop by cooking it into soups, stews, and sauces. Or go further and try freezing, pickling, root cellaring, drying, or fermenting it. Another solution is to split a share with a friend, something I've done because I wanted less food so I could enjoy my garden but still reap the benefits of my CSA membership. (For creative ways to use your CSA bounty, see page 62.)

Are you willing to share the risk? The original premise of CSAs was that the members would share the risk of farming as well as the bounty. As Robyn Van En, cofounder of the North American CSA movement, puts it, "The risk of getting no crop is extremely slight. The risk of getting half of all crops is slight. The risk of getting half of any one crop is good. The risk of getting 75 percent of some crops and 125 percent of some others is excellent."

Crops may come in as expected, but one year the berry harvest might be scant while the tomatoes are plentiful. Members take a portion of what's harvested, sharing the good and bad years with the farmer — no refunds are forthcoming. (To boost their odds of surviving, some farms do operate on a strict share basis and give their members a set amount of food, which is usually generous, then sell some vegetables, especially bumper crops, elsewhere.)

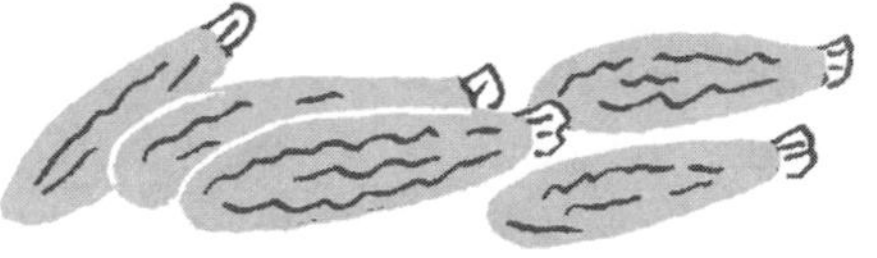

GET IT DIRECT

ADVANTAGES OF JOINING A CSA

- **Fabulous food.** You'll receive healthful, organic or sustainably raised food that is freshly harvested for you each week.
- **A more healthful diet.** You're likely to eat more vegetables, the one piece of diet advice agreed on for 100 years. They'll be fresh and sustainably raised, too!
- **On-the-farm perks.** These might include pick-your-own fruit or flowers, or a la carte farm items such as eggs, bread, or maple syrup.
- **Idyllic outings.** It's so much fun, you (and your family) won't realize it's educational.
- **New experiences.** You'll have the chance to cook and enjoy new foods, always at peak freshness.
- **A sense of community.** You'll get to know your farmer and fellow farm-share members on harvest days and at events.
- **Land stewardship.** You will be directly supporting sustainable management of the land in your region.

• **A connection to nature.** You'll gain an understanding of the flow of growing seasons, learn about how your food is grown firsthand, and connect with the land it's grown on.

• **A chance to boost future farms.** CSAs fulfill an essential gap by training young farm apprentices, a venture worthy of your support.

Origins of the CSA Movement

The North American CSA movement started in New England in 1985 at two farms: Temple-Wilton Community Farm in New Hampshire and Indian Line Farm in Massachusetts. Robyn Van En and Jan Vander Tuin spearheaded the North American CSA movement from Indian Line Farm. They were jump-started by Susan Witt, of the nearby E.F. Schumacher Society, an organization committed to local economies. Soon, Robyn was spreading the gospel to other farms and receiving so many calls from intrigued farmers that she wrote *Basic Formula to Create Community Supported Agriculture* by hand in 1988, copied it, and for $2, mailed it to farmers who requested it. The book inspired a generation of farmers.

BRING A CSA SHARE TO YOUR WORKPLACE

Organizing workplace CSAs is a great way to boost a local farm and bring better food to your place of business. Download a how-to manual by following the link to CISA in Resources.

HOW TO FIND A CSA NEAR YOU

CSA farms are located everywhere. To find one near you, follow the link for the Robyn Van En Center in Resources.

THE CSA TODAY

In 2008 the Robyn Van En Center at Wilson College in Chambersburg, Pennsylvania, estimated that 1,700 to 2,000 CSAs operate in North America. They vary widely in style and scope, including smaller Northeast farms where Robyn's concept of active core members flourish, to Midwest CSAs that are more farmer-driven and may even be multifarm operations, to gigantic CSAs in California. Additionally, other ingredient- and buyer-specific CSAs have sprung up, such as meat or restaurant CSAs, sometimes called buying clubs (see page 68).

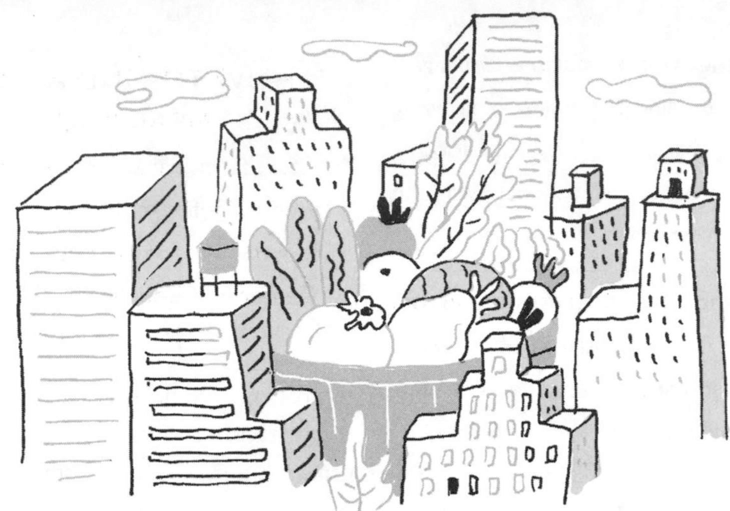

The Modern CSA: Two Case Studies

CONNECTING CITY DWELLERS WITH CSAs — JUST FOOD IN NYC

Just Food's CSA program in New York City started in 1995 with a conference to develop CSAs that would bring regional farm foods to community members. By the following year, six new city CSAs were in full swing, each with an individual drop point independently run by its own core members. Still growing, they facilitated 24 farms, averaging 100 miles from NYC, servicing 62 CSA drop points throughout the city. The smallest had 20 member shares in Harlem, Manhattan, and the largest had 200 shares in Cobble Hill, Brooklyn.

Just Food makes the farm match, provides CSA education and technical support, and holds annual conferences. Organizing these city drop-point CSAs requires more than one person, so people get to know each other and a social network often evolves. Paula Lukats, program manager, says she's met more people in the three years she's been a member of the Williamsburg Green Point, Brooklyn CSA than in the 15 years she's lived in her neighborhood!

While some are simply pick-up spots, most city CSAs arrange farm visits and some hold potlucks. One screens films; another holds yoga classes. In Astoria, the CSA holds once-a-month nutrition classes and is planning a block party to raise funds for low-income shares.

A COLLEGE CSA

Becky Davis, a college junior, is looking forward to the first share of her eight-week CSA membership, which promises to be a bag of eight or so items, including a head of lettuce, cabbage, or bunches of beets. Members also have optional ingredients for purchase, brought in from other farms, including honey, meat, milk, and yogurt.

Becky is one of a growing number of students who have rejected campus food in favor of the real stuff, in this case farm-fresh food from Norwich Meadows Farm in Binghamton, New York. Norwich Meadows makes six stops in New York City, including New York University. Some schools, like Vassar, are taking the concept even further with a CSA farm on campus serving low-income households.

Becky's Morningside Heights CSA is administered by student coordinator Megan McNally and a school club, The Columbia University Food Sustainability Project. The project also manages a community garden and works to green the campus in other ways. "Food is tangential to so many issues and areas of study that we attract a wide array of people, beyond environmental studies, which was the original core of students," says Becky, who is copresident of the club. (For more information on local food on campus, follow the link for the Real Food Challenge in Resources.)

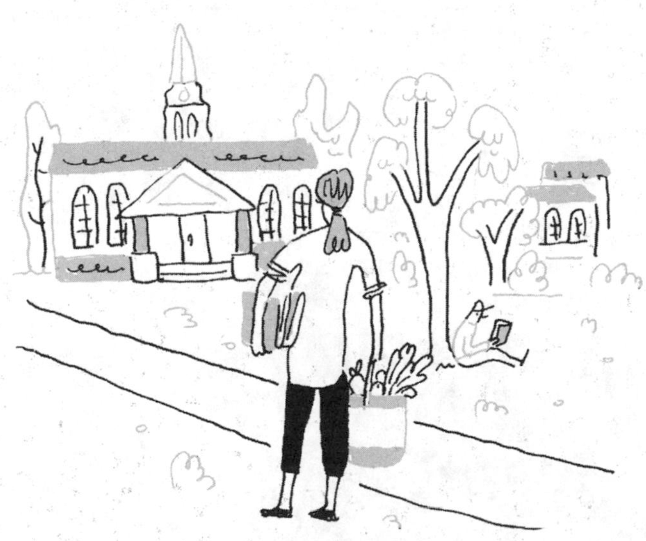

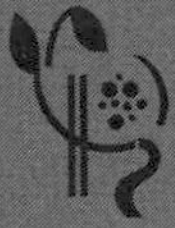

The CSA Connection

"Being in a city, CSA reconnects us to the land. I love having a connection to a farm I can visit and feel a part of, knowing my farmer (and asking him all my garden questions), and believing that each vegetable I pick up is truly what he tells me it is — because I can see it for myself. The best part, though, is that I hardly ever enter a grocery store anymore! I receive all my veggies, meat, and dairy from my CSA, so it is very convenient."

STACY ORNSTEIN

Astoria CSA member, Queens, New York
(matched with her neighborhood CSA through Just Food)

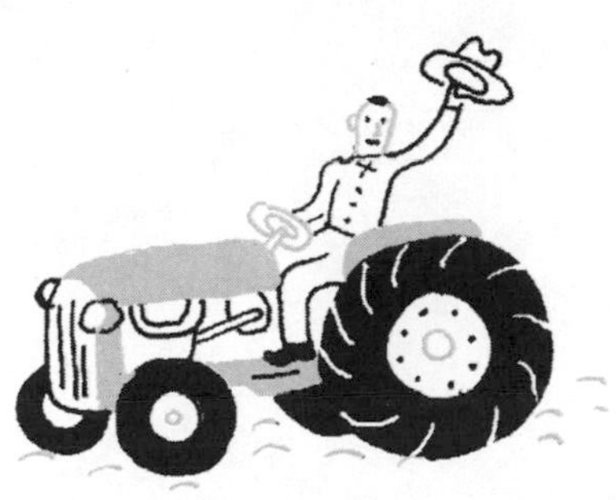

Spoutwood Farm CSA

"On harvest day there's such abundance. You get to talk with other members, swapping tales and sharing recipes. The kids grew up there. My daughter, who grew up and moved to the city, still likes to come out to the farm. It shaped her life, and she now runs community gardens in Brooklyn. She buys her food from a farmers' market and food co-ops. She brought that spirit from here to her city life."

LIZ LEINWAND

Working member, Spoutwood CSA, Baltimore, Maryland

Spoutwood Farm sits in a hollow with two streams running through it, just 45 minutes north of Baltimore, Maryland. Rising from the water are two hills (Frodo's Hill is named for its hobbitlike straw bale building), and nestled between them is an 1857 brick farmhouse. Out front, three acres of intensively farmed vegetables feed 100 member families.

The 26-acre farm has been a CSA for 13 years, but it is also an educational nonprofit, hosting seasonal festivals that are attended by 300 revelers who camp in tents on the second hill. Its School of Sustainable Living holds classes on topics like preserving the harvest and beekeeping, as well as a star-gazing observatory program. Farmer Rob Wood, who got

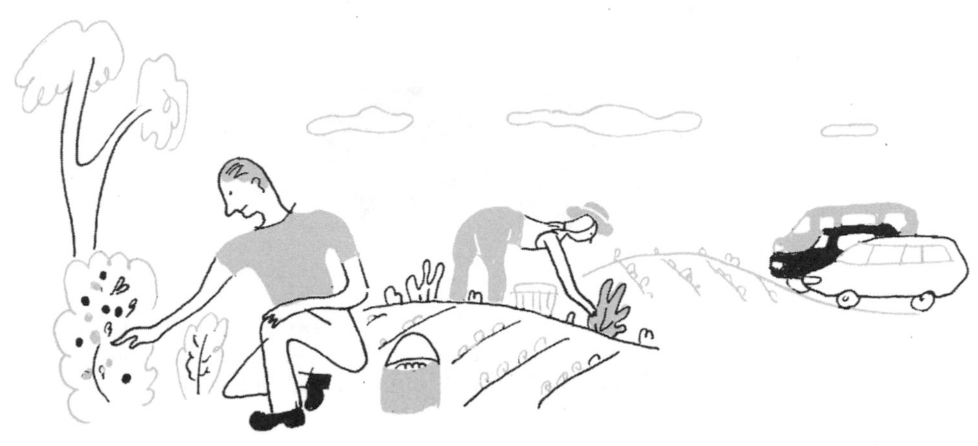

the urge to farm while working in the Peace Corps in India, sees farming as a way to introduce visitors to nature. He prides himself on the farm's easy interplay of cultivated and wild land. "The farm is very green with lots of wildlife," he says.

Rob calls his CSA the "crowning jewel" of Spoutwood Farm. Most of the farm's crops are harvested the day members pick up their shares. Harvest starts at about 5:30 AM with this year's apprentices Zach, Dana, and Derrick working until 8 or 9 AM when working members, who barter labor for CSA shares, join them. By midmorning, as many as 15 people are harvesting crops and talking among themselves, most focusing on individual vegetables or herbs. A few members assemble weekly bouquets of flowers in the field, one person ferrying food to the distribution area. By noon everything is harvested and trucks depart for their drop-off points.

Later that day, 30 members pick up their shares by the farm's house, easily assembling as many as 10 to 15 different kinds of vegetables and herbs per share, all of which are posted on a menu board. The remaining 70 or so members, who mostly receive prebagged shares, pick up at drop points in Baltimore, the Northern Baltimore area, and York, Pennsylvania, about 20 minutes away. Shares include 22 weeks of organically grown vegetables, on-farm workshops, and a members' party. And in an effort to support neighboring farms and make the CSA more of a one-stop shop, Rob has introduced popular add-on shares in meat, dairy (milk, cheese, and eggs), and bread.

Spoutwood incorporates a strong educational component to its shares, providing numerous tools for its members to better understand and use the harvest. Offerings include week-by-week harvest information, online recipes, and a 60-page membership book offering in-depth information on each vegetable, along with additional recipes. This insight is particularly helpful to new members who may be unfamiliar with some of Rob's crops.

When I spoke with Rob in mid-July, the week's shares included lettuce, scallions, kale, beets, potatoes, green peppers, cucumbers, summer squash, green beans, cabbage, broccoli or cauliflower, garlic, oregano, and a bouquet of flowers. That week, he let members know that tomatoes and eggplant were coming in late. He also informed them that he reluctantly sprayed their kale on Tuesday with *pyganic*, an organic substance, nontoxic to humans and made from chrysanthemums, which breaks down in

ORGANIC?

Like many CSAs, Spoutwood Farm uses organic methods but is not certified organic. And like many sustainable farmers, working to replenish rather than deplete their farm's natural resources, Rob finds the certification process prohibitively expensive. He feels that his methods, practiced before certification became government domain, are the best proof of his operation's commitment to building the soil naturally. They also provide an environment for the humane treatment of animals, and avoid the use of toxic substances.

12 to 24 hours. Although pick-up was on Thursday, he advised members to wash their kale thoroughly.

CSAs attract all types, but Spoutwood's members tend to be health-conscious baby boomers and young people with kids. Last year, a couple joined the CSA while starting an exercise program and dropped 100 pounds between them. Now, farm visits are part of their routine. Members also round up their friends. This season, one go-getter signed up 10 new CSA members from her synagogue's congregation in Baltimore, creating a new drop-off point for Rob.

Rob says his best members have grown into a way of eating that involves the farm, and they can't wait for the next season. His biggest surprises come from the vegetables themselves, such as kale and chard, not favorites at first, but members soon find great ways to use them. Kohlrabi, a crisp cultivar in the cabbage family, garnered some suspicious

WAYS TO MAKE THE MOST OF YOUR CSA BOUNTY

1. Listen to your mom: include more vegetables in your diet.
2. Learn to cook and savor familiar and unfamiliar vegetables.
3. Eat at home more; cook more.
4. Share harvest meals with friends and family.
5. Throw a party!
6. Only take home what you'll really use (even if it's less than your share).
7. Give some away to those who need it. (See page 52 for more suggestions.)
8. Make extra to eat later in the week; freeze, can, or dry.

looks at first from young member Danny Snyder, but he now calls it his favorite vegetable.

But sometimes, especially at the height of the season when there's lots of food coming in, people get overwhelmed. While the recipes help, Rob warns members to be patient, not to expect that their CSA membership will instantly change how they relate to food. Rather, he tells them, it's more of a lifestyle change that happens incrementally.

Rob and his wife, Lucy, particularly enjoy the transformative nature the farm has on children. And both are filled with stories about kids. Two involved boys, one an Indian immigrant, who recognized the okra — a vegetable he remembered fondly from his country but had never seen here, either growing or on a plate. The other was a boy who picked carrots for the first time, pulling the magical orange vegetable from the soil and keeping it under his pillow for 2 weeks, not allowing anyone to touch it.

"When you see kids make the connection you know that is going to stay with them for life," Rob says.

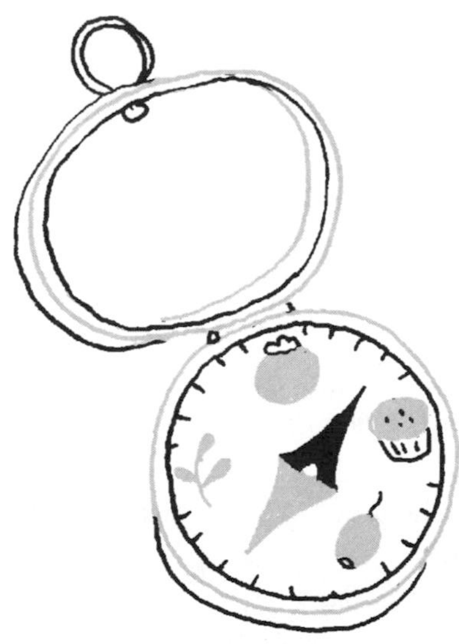

Spoutwood Farm's Weekly Share List

Below is a sample CSA weekly share list, to give you a general idea of the array of vegetables and how they change over the season. Of course, CSA shares vary by climate, crop, and number of weeks; some CSAs also have winter shares. Each CSA has its own style, too. Spoutwood Farm includes lettuces or lettuce mix and a bouquet of flowers each week. It also offers add-on shares of bread, meat, dairy, eggs, and cheese. Because it uses lots of volunteers and barters shares for work, it doesn't have pick-your-own crops.

WEEK 1	Peas, arugula, bok choy, green onions, mint, oregano, radishes
WEEK 2	Mustard greens, garlic scapes, greens, bok choy, green onions ASSORTMENT VARIES BY DROP-OFF LOCATION, BUT MAY INCLUDE: green onions, radishes, Swiss chard, kohlrabi, mint, oregano
WEEK 3	SAME AS WEEK 2 PLUS: kale, mizuna (a peppery green), Chinese cabbage, broccoli, cilantro
WEEK 4	SAME AS WEEK 3 PLUS: lettuce mix (mesclun), endive, beets, collard greens, purple basil
WEEK 5	SAME AS WEEK 4 PLUS: radicchio, carrots ASSORTMENT BY DROP-OFF LOCATION INCLUDES: cabbage, cauliflower, burgundy beans, basil, dill
WEEK 6	Green onions, broccoli, beets, carrots, green peppers, collard greens ASSORTMENT BY DROP-OFF LOCATION INCLUDES: cabbage, burgundy beans, cucumbers, basil, Thai basil

WEEK 7	Green onions, kale, beets, potatoes, green peppers, cucumbers, summer squash and zucchini, green beans ASSORTMENT BY DROP-OFF LOCATION INCLUDES: cabbage, broccoli or cauliflower, garlic, oregano
WEEK 8	Varieties of tomatoes, eggplant, Swiss chard, green onions, potatoes, green peppers, cucumbers, summer squash and zucchini, and green, yellow, and burgundy beans ASSORTMENT BY DROP-OFF LOCATION INCLUDES: cabbage, cauliflower, garlic, basil
WEEK 9	Varieties of tomatoes, eggplant, kale, green onions, potatoes, green peppers, cucumbers, varieties of summer squash and zucchini, sage, apple mint
WEEK 10	SAME AS WEEK 9 PLUS: Swiss chard and collard greens instead of kale, Anaheim peppers, basil instead of sage
WEEK 11	Varieties of tomatoes, eggplant, Swiss chard, red and yellow onions, potatoes, green peppers, Anaheim peppers, habanero peppers, cucumbers, varieties of summer squash and zucchini, Thai basil, sage CSA potluck and core meeting
WEEK 12	Varieties of tomatoes, eggplant, collard greens, kale, beans, potatoes, green peppers, hot paper lantern peppers, cucumbers, varieties of summer squash including zucchini, garlic, basil
WEEK 13	Varieties of tomatoes, red and yellow onions, eggplant, green peppers, hot paper lantern peppers, varieties of summer squash including zucchini, Swiss chard, young mizuna (a peppery green), oregano, basil, green and purple beans (for some)
WEEK 14	Varieties of tomatoes, red and yellow onions, carrots, potatoes, green peppers, hot paper lantern peppers, green and burgundy beans, a variety of summer squash including zucchini, kale, arugula, spinach garlic, basil, sage

WEEK 15	Varieties of tomatoes (now dwindling), acorn squash, leeks, eggplant varieties, radishes, green and purple beans, green peppers, hot paper lantern peppers, Swiss chard, collard greens, rosemary, basil
WEEK 16	Varieties of tomatoes and multicolored green-red peppers (both radically dwindling now), radishes, hot paper lantern peppers, Chinese cabbage, bok choy, yellow onions, potatoes, arugula, kohlrabi, basil, Thai basil
WEEK 17	Eggplant (the last), chestnuts (from a neighboring farm), multicolored green-red peppers (radically dwindling now), hot paper lantern peppers, carrots, kohlrabi, arugula, mizuna, spinach, collard greens, bok choy, rosemary, Thai basil
WEEK 18	Organic apples (from a neighboring farm), beets, leeks, radishes, tomatoes (very few), hot paper lantern peppers, kohlrabi, broccoli, Swiss chard, arugula, mustard greens, bok choy, sage, apple mint
WEEK 19	Beets, last of the green-red peppers, Anaheim peppers, kohlrabi, broccoli, cauliflower, Swiss chard, arugula, mustard greens, onions, thyme, oregano
WEEK 20	Sweet potatoes, turnips, beets, cabbage, the last green peppers, Anaheim and hot paper lantern peppers, broccoli, cauliflower, collard greens, watermelon (from a neighboring organic farm), onions, sage
WEEK 21	Chinese cabbage, butternut squash, spinach, beets, broccoli, cauliflower, arugula, turnips, onions, rosemary
WEEK 22	Butternut squash, beets, turnips, cabbage (3 varieties to choose from), mustard greens, mizuna, beets, collard greens, kale

Buying Clubs

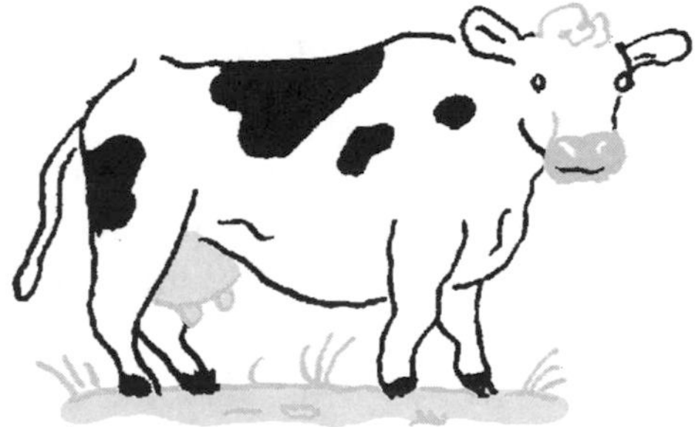

"Our buying club is an ideal way to have access to food we couldn't get otherwise and to support a local dairy."

TRICE ATCHISON

Member of The Milk House Raw Milk Club, Alford, Massachusetts

Locavores nationwide are initiating buying clubs by forging direct farm-to-consumer relationships to procure farm-fresh ingredients. Buying club members unite to purchase better quality or hard-to-find foods, such as raw milk or sustainably raised meat, while helping to keep a rancher or dairy farmer in business. Food is purchased collectively, in a large group order, which sometimes allows for a discount over retail prices. Then, it's delivered to a location that's convenient to club members, usually once a month or sometimes once a week.

Clubs may be started by the producer, but just as often they're initiated by community members in search of quality farm food, sometimes at a discount. They organize the club in partnership with one farm, then volunteer to keep the club going once it's set up, limiting infrastructure to a bare minimum. Rules vary; some clubs require minimal membership fees or minimum orders.

Buying clubs are not new; consumers have always chipped in together to buy better-quality or cheaper food. Decades ago, I was a member of one of the many "natural food clubs," which later morphed into food co-ops. Many of their foods, including then-hard-to-find beans and grains, are now easy to spot in specialty stores and even supermarkets. This simple system works well for group purchases of any kind, so necessity has shifted the focus to hard-to-procure local foods, like raw milk and sustainably produced meat.

Raw Milk

Raw milk is unhomogenized whole milk (cream on the top) called "raw" because it is unpasteurized. Some controversy surrounds raw milk's safety and health benefits, but not its flavor, which is superior, with a real dairy taste few of us remember. There's a demand for fresh, local, raw milk, and buying clubs fill that need.

Pros. Proponents strongly feel that raw milk from grass-fed cows (as opposed to those raised on feedlots) contains

WHERE DO I GET RAW MILK?

State laws vary on the sale of raw milk. Currently only a handful of states allow its sale in retail stores. In other states, raw milk must be purchased on the farm. For state laws, to find raw milk clubs near you, and more, follow the Real Milk link to A Campaign for Real Milk in Resources.

more nutrients, as well as healthful bacteria and enzymes that are normally killed during pasteurization.

Another pro is what raw milk *doesn't* contain: growth hormones and antibiotics. Raw milk producers tend to be sustainable farmers, so drinkers enjoy supporting local eco-friendly farms that preserve our working landscape and treat their animals humanely. They also insist that the safety standards for processing raw milk are much higher than those on large-scale agribusiness dairy farms, where illnesses have been tied to unpasteurized milk.

FOR THE SAKE OF FLAVOR

Raya Ariella, buying club organizer, uses freshness as the criteria for comparing the flavor of raw and conventional milk — the same as fresh versus frozen or canned corn, or bread made from freshly milled whole wheat as opposed to fluffy, white, supermarket bread. And, of course, the milk of each herd has its own flavor, unlike conventional milk, which generally combines milk from countless cows.

Cons. On the negative side, I defer to respected nutritionist Marion Nestle, who writes with clarity and good sense about food but does not drink raw milk. She believes raw milk can quite possibly be consumed safely and that it does taste better. But she says the nutritional benefits are minimal, if they exist at all. More importantly, she doesn't feel consuming raw milk is worth the risk of illness from some of the "bad" bacteria that would ordinarily be killed during pasteurization.

MY LOCAL MILK CLUB

My local club, The Milk House Raw Milk Club, is only a few years old with 40 members but aims to work its way up to 100 members, which will provide a good living for the farmer, Paul Paisley, who farms on rented land.

His farm is in a rural area, and most members know Paul, either from town or from the annual members' party. He just wants to milk the cows, so he leaves the organization to Raya, the club's manager. (He says the cows are the club's stars, not him.) Paul has a license from the Massachusetts Department of Agricultural Resources to sell his raw milk to consumers. He also wholesales milk to local cheese maker, Michael Miller, who makes Berkshire Blue Cheese.

During the cold months, Paul's cows graze on pasture at Twin Oaks

SHARES GALORE

Cow shares for meat or milk allow consumers to collectively own a cow, in order to have a reliable source of raw milk and natural meat. In some cases, several families own a cow together and share the costs and labor related to maintaining it. In other cases, individuals may buy shares of a cow from a farmer in exchange for a weekly supply of milk.

Farm in stunning Alford, a town in the Berkshire hills of western Massachusetts. In the winter, they're fed hay cut from those pastures along with grain grown up-county on the Wirtes Farm in Lanesborough.

The pick-up point is the local co-op, where they can't sell raw milk (it's illegal) or even exchange money for the club. They simply provide a fridge near the registers for club members. My first jug of milk was waiting there as prearranged.

I doubt anyone will dispute the flavor of raw milk. It is far superior to pasteurized milk, with a more distinctive milky flavor, which is variable, depending on what the cows have eaten. My milk had a very slightly orange cast, as if the sun were captured in the jug. The top one-quarter to one-third was a whiter, dense cream, which can be decanted for its own use or, as is common, shaken up for whole milk.

The club works simply. An annual membership fee covers any small administrative expenses, including Raya's time. (Fees vary from club to club; some clubs operated by farmers or their family members don't have an annual fee.) Milk is often sold off the farm or brought to a drop-off point, generally once or twice a week.

Meat-Buying Clubs

Convenient, affordable, sustainably raised meat can be difficult to find. Because of this, meat-buying clubs (sometimes called meat CSAs) are springing up all over the country. This meat is often raised for its flavor rather than for its ability to fatten quickly and withstand the inhumane conditions often found in confined animal feeding operations (CAFOs).

Demand for sustainably raised meat has increased for several reasons, including the realization that large animals are at the top of the food chain

The Meat-Eaters Club

"As a family, we enjoy beef, pork, and lamb, and our dog loves the bones! Cooking with grass-fed meat was a challenge at first — we had some pretty tough steaks in the beginning — but only because it is much leaner and needs to be cooked less. During the summer I make flank steak and kebab meat. In fall and winter I cook a lot of roasts and stews, and the flavor is amazing. I am now to the point where I will set a recipe aside if I don't have the cut of meat I need.

I remember a moment after our first delivery when I got an overwhelming feeling that what we were doing was really awesome. We were not only helping to support a great family farm, but we were succeeding in feeding our family healthy, safe meat and enabling others to do the same. It was a real sense of community."

MEGHAN MAGONEGIL

West Seattle Meat-Eaters Buying Club, Seattle, Washington

If you buy part of an animal, find out the net weight first and make sure you have freezer space, as the meat will likely come to you frozen. You know what a pound of burger meat looks like, so just multiply up. You'll be amazed at what you can fit in.

and thus contain more toxins, a process called biomagnification. Considerable alarm about the treatment of feedlot animals and ecological concerns about grain-gobbling cows are also growing. And on the flip side, recent research has revealed the health benefits from the fatty acids like conjugated linoleic acid (CLA) in grass-fed animals (see page 75). Still, USDA-approved slaughterhouses, as well as sustainable farmers and ranchers, can be few and far between, so making the arrangements for a meat-buying club, which takes the cow from pasture to table, can be a challenge.

Of course, it's easiest to join an existing club, but if one isn't around, there are many ways to get one going. You can start by finding a willing farmer through venues where he already sells his meat, such as farmers' markets, farm stands, and food co-ops. Or you may hear about a butcher collaborating with a farmer. All this might take a bit of investigation, but if it's the only way to find sustainably raised meat, go for it. It paid off for me in unforgettable farm-cured bacon, grass-fed burgers, and more. For more information on starting your own meat-buying club, follow the link to The Ethicurean in Resources.

AD HOC MEAT-BUYING CLUBS

My local meat-buying club isn't really a club at all. Since I have no established club near me and our farms are generally too small to set them up, I use more of an ad hoc arrangement. Through word of mouth or the farmers' market, I find a farm that raises meat animals sustainably, and then I e-mail around to see who's interested in buying some. Usually, a friend and I agree to split a quarter cow or whole hog (some of it smoked), each of which provides about 100 pounds of meat. Or I buy a lamb on my own, which nets about 25 pounds.

Thundering Hooves Meat-Buying Club

"Our environmental philosophy is that Nature knows best. For thousands of years, multiple species of animals grazed unplowed fields of clovers and grasses. The sod held the moisture, the clovers added nitrogen for the grasses, the animals recycled the plants, and the microorganisms rejoiced! This was and is sustainable agriculture."

JOEL HUESBY

Thundering Hooves, Walla Walla Valley, Washington

Thundering Hooves is a farm and meat store in the Walla Walla Valley, Washington, serving 25 regional meat-buying clubs. Along with other meat-buying clubs across the country, Thundering Hooves has developed an easy way for members to purchase clean meat that's sustainably and humanely raised and slaughtered.

HOW IT WORKS

A look at Thundering Hooves' setup may just encourage you to join a meat-buying club or start your own!

At Thundering Hooves customers sign up on their Web site — which is filled with meat-related information — place orders, and select one of the club's monthly drop spots. A cost estimate for grass-fed beef, pork, lamb, or chicken by cut is available four days in advance; the final price is e-mailed two days later, after the meat is weighed, along with a pick-up reminder. These days the average order is about $80, but an order can be much smaller, as long as the group meets the minimum (or at least tries; they are lenient). Customers pay when the truck rolls in once a month, delivering frozen meat packages labeled with each member's name. Pickup is essential — no one likes to have defrosting meat sitting in his or her driveway! — but if customers forget, they get a reminder call from Keith Swanson, farm family member and the driver. Any meat that isn't picked up is sold to other members.

Usually, the clubs are managed by a hostess, who fields queries from interested consumers, solicits members, and allows the truck to park for half an hour in her driveway once a month. In exchange for this minimal amount of work, the hostess gets a discount on the meat.

AN EPIPHANY AND REBIRTH

This year Thundering Hooves, a fourth-generation farm, is processing 350 head of cattle — some of it from other local farms — on a total of 625 owned and leased acres. Many farms like Thundering Hooves survived until the "green revolution" after World War II. At that point, illogical farm subsidies, with their promises of higher yield and lower prices, helped farm income to plummet.

In 1994, family member Joel Huesby decided to fight this downward spiral and work toward a profitable, sustainable farm with a variety of animals — cattle, chickens, turkeys, goats, sheep, and pigs — all raised on open pasture rather than in confined feedlots. The herds are moved every 4 to 5 days, giving the pastures time to recycle nutrients. The cattle calmly follow the truck — even the sound of a voice — to the next pasture. Huesby doesn't use antibiotics indiscriminately and doesn't give animals hormones to boost their growth. All of these practices lead to more contented animals and healthier meats.

In 2004 the family's new incarnation, Thundering Hooves, bought a meat shop and, in 2006, a USDA-approved slaughterhouse. That same year the company began selling meat to restaurant clients, who learned of the farm by word of mouth and came in droves. In 2007, the family launched their first meat-buying club, and within a year and a half,

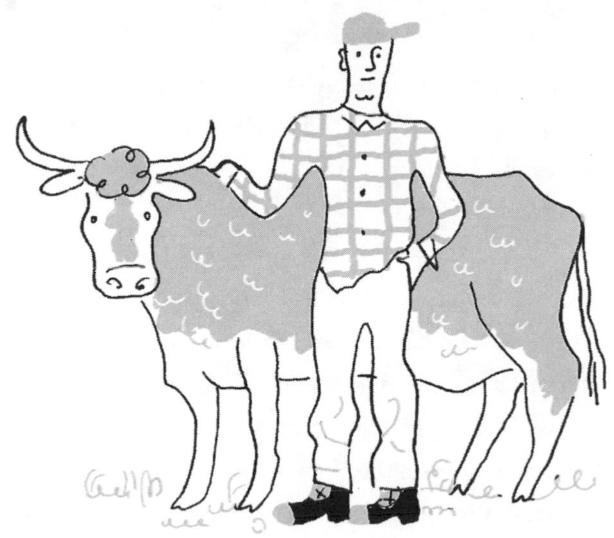

they were supporting 25 regional meat-buying clubs with as many as 200 members and individual buyers. Today one-third of their business comes from their Walla Walla shop, one-third from restaurants, and one-third from buying clubs. Thundering Hooves expects to double its buying club membership in a year or two. Demand for sustainably raised meat is moderate in the immediate region but is high in Portland and Seattle. The buying clubs meet that demand.

GRASS-FED AND PASTURE-RAISED CATTLE

When people ask what grass fed-and-finished meat tastes like, Keith Swanson of Thundering Hooves tells them it's stronger and richer tasting, that most people like it, but that it isn't for everyone. "It's real beef flavor," he says.

It takes skill to raise tender grass-fed meat. Farmers raising animals on pasture have to be patient because more time is needed to fatten them on grass than grain, and fattened animals produce tender meat.

The end results depend on factors consumers can't control, like the breed and age of the cow, method of slaughtering, and importantly, the quality of the grass (which is why many ranchers who raise cattle this way call themselves "grass farmers"). The bottom line is that the farmers have to know what they are doing and set high standards for their grass-fed meat, or the meat will be tough.

While grass-fed-and-finished beef can be world class and eye opening when it comes to taste, it doesn't have the same kind of marbleized fat many of us are used to and so requires more attention during cooking. Less plentiful tender cuts, like filet, should be seared and served rare or medium-rare. Less tender cuts are better braised or roasted slowly, but not too long. (To braise, sear on the outside, then cook covered with a few cups of liquid — wine, tomatoes, or broth — and seasonings.) Burger can be cooked as usual, and grass-fed burger is extremely flavorful, delicious, and distinctive.

Note that many farms finish pasture-raised animals on a little to a lot of grain for a more familiar flavor and to increase marbleized fat for tenderness. So if you can't find grass-fed-and-finished meat, look for pasture-raised meat finished minimally on local grain and, when possible, sustainably raised.

Stores of All Kinds

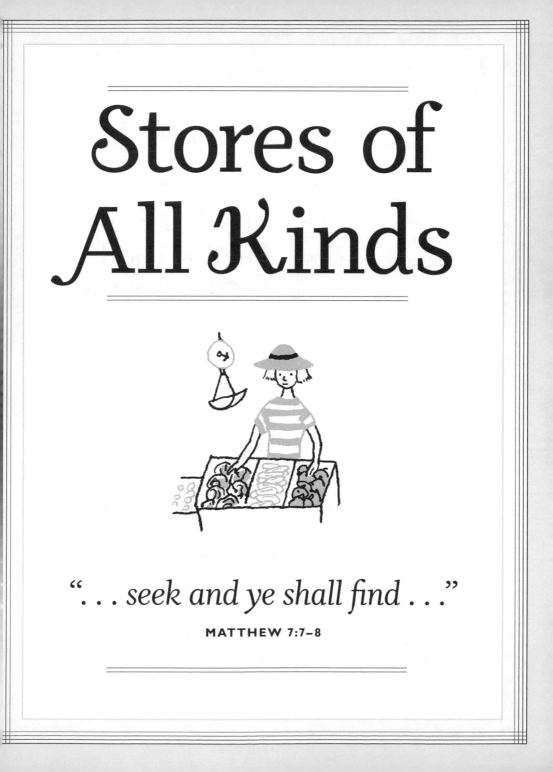

". . . seek and ye shall find . . ."

MATTHEW 7:7–8

Though direct-from-the-farm shopping is the most straightforward way to buy local food, you're probably not going to stop shopping at retail stores anytime soon, especially supermarkets, so you might as well become a smart shopper.

Finding local food at retail stores has its own level of satisfaction, both from hunting and from discovering the treasure. But you'll need to hone your local food detective skills and develop your fortitude, because although you may spot some local ingredients quickly, it's likely to take a little time and patience to uncover others. Eventually, though, one find will lead to the next and you'll be adding favorite discoveries to your local food inventory for your next shopping trip. And if you channel your inner shopper, it's even easier. Imagine the joy you take in tracking down a great pair of shoes. Now make the switch in your head and approach finding local food in the same way.

Retailers are in a position to change the face of farming by buying locally. It's more work for them because they have to buy from more producers, so encourage them by praising their good work when you find it!

The Basics of Finding Local Food Anywhere

I've lived in all kinds of places: I grew up in the suburbs, spent a chunk of my life in the city, and ended up in the country. But no single location had a lock on easy procurement of local foods. And within each location, I found fabulous local food in both expected and unexpected places — including the best local goat cheese

INDIRECT SHOPPING FOR LOCAL FARM FOOD

When you're out buying shampoo, why not nose around for locally grown, raised, or produced food? This task can be daunting because our national food system isn't set up to feature local foods. But be patient, relax, and maintain your sense of humor, and soon you'll be integrating the hunt for local food into your everyday life.

Foraging for local food is harder than shopping off a list. But even small finds have enormous payback as you accumulate lasting sources of fabulous food. See it as a life-long adventure. Watch and encourage positive changes.

imaginable, which I found in a liquor store.

BEFORE YOU SHOP

Make your life easier by doing a little homework first. Seek out anyone you know who is passionate about food. Look for ads, articles, and Web sites that clue you in to businesses that invest in local food. Pick up an Edible Communities publication or other independently owned, regionally focused magazine in your area. Local food initiatives or national organizations like Slow Food may also give you leads.

And of course, *go to the source.* If you're already shopping directly from farmers, they'll tell you whether they sell off-farm and, if so, where. A regional farm that's too far to patronize on a regular basis may sell at the supermarket. A green bean producer you've met at a farmers' market may also supply the local food co-op. A vineyard can steer you to liquor stores where their wines are sold. My local cheese maker gave me a list of her clients, so when I couldn't get down to the farm, I could still buy her cheese.

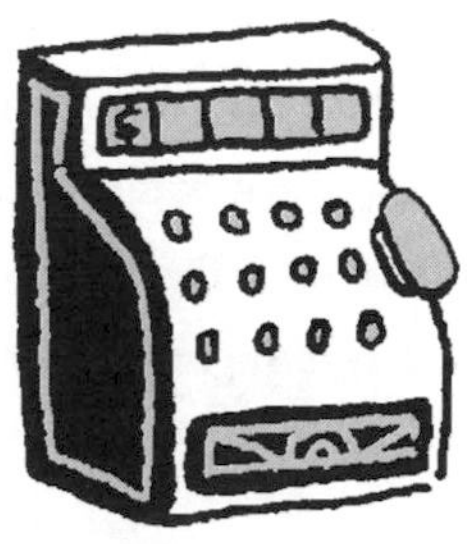

LOCAL FOOD MANTRA: ASK

The first rule is to ask, "What's local?" wherever you shop. Don't be shy. And of course, if you don't know who the buyer is, use the mantra again: ask. We all like to talk about our work, and professional food buyers are no exception. They're generally courteous even when they don't have a clue where their food comes from. If they don't know, they may be able to find out, and sometimes that's as easy as checking the label on a box in the storeroom. Besides, you may have sparked their interest. The next time you go shopping, they may have better answers. And asking creates demand.

DEVELOP A RELATIONSHIP WITH THE FOOD BUYER

This relationship can't be overstated. At any retail store, learn who the food buyer is and let him or her know you are interested in buying local foods. Over time this small action will reap more benefits than all the detective work in the world.

START WITH PRODUCE . . .

. . . then try whole foods, and finally value-added products. Although notable exceptions abound, produce is the local food you're most likely to find at stores. Read labels. Ask. Move on from there to other whole foods, which are those that are consumed as close to their natural state as possible:

- Milk, not low-fat pudding
- Carrots, not carrot-mango juice
- Honey, not honey cake
- Maple syrup, not maple-flavored cereal

When local food is processed into value-added products, it is more likely to be processed the old-fashioned way: milk into ice cream, maple syrup into maple candy, grapes into wine or jelly. Traditional kinds of processing generally use fewer ingredients and less junk, a healthful by-product of local products.

READ SIGNS, BUT ALSO LOOK BEYOND THEM

Fortunately, more signage these days will steer you to local foods. Look for required country of origin labeling (COOL) to tell you if your food was shipped in from elsewhere. If you see consumer information that tells you where the food was grown — name of farm and location, not just country — praise it. Try not to settle for vague terms like "native" or even "local," but ask specifically *where* the food is from.

BECOME A LOCAL FOOD SIGN RETAIL LOBBYIST

Work on getting better signage in place. Start by asking the food buyer, such as the produce manager, for it. If you shop at a large chain where signage needs to be cleared with corporate headquarters, ask for an address and phone number, then make the request. You can do this solo (or with a petition) by letter and a follow-up call, but you're most likely to get action by working with a local organization that promotes agriculture. Your partnership will let them know that the community is behind the request and will include farmers in the process. Be persistent. It's worked for me, although I had to print my own signs to supermarket specifications and have them laminated. (Save copies, because after they come down each season, they tend to disappear.) Don't be disappointed if you don't see immediate action. Every request is registered and can ultimately change buying and labeling policies.

Unfortunately, signage can be not only misleading but also downright inaccurate. This misinformation happens a lot when, for instance, stores don't keep up with the turnover in the produce section; local food signs often remain when bins are refilled with food from Argentina or some other faraway place.

Develop a sense of store policy through your questions. Look beyond surface observations. Get to know

Expert Advice

LEARN FROM YOUR RETAIL PRODUCE MANAGER OR STAFF

Joe Deluca, a hearty-looking New Englander in his late thirties, has worked in retail produce for 20 years and has watched it grow from a long, single supermarket aisle to a riot of rows bursting with seasonless food from every corner of the planet.

I stopped in after walking past a new sign hawking local foods in front of the market. I asked him what was local, as nothing was blatantly marked as such. Some local items, like the corn, had gone by, but the butternut squash and apples were still available, packed in bags with their Connecticut farm name. Joe mentioned that the plastic-bagged apples were regional, too, but they simply had the store logo on them, so there was no way of knowing. He pointed out some cut vegetables from the Pioneer Valley (about 60 miles away), whose packaging also bore a farm name. And, as he was bringing out collards stiff with freshness, he noted that they, too, were organically grown in the Pioneer Valley. I never would have known if he hadn't mentioned it, though their tiny metal tie had a farm name in tiny letters.

Local produce sections that make things easy for consumers are rare, but clear signage would have sold it fast. I made a mental note to call or write corporate headquarters, but the lesson is to look carefully and ask, ask, ask.

As I was leaving, Joe told me that shoppers are angry when they see that some of the produce isn't local, but they also insist on eating whatever they want all year long.

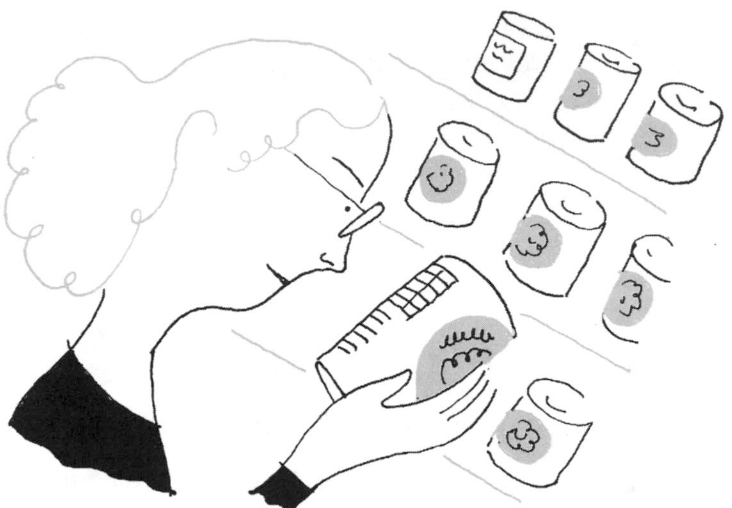

the food buyer over time. *Everyone's jumping on the local food bandwagon, and we're all responsible if we don't hold retailers accountable for accuracy in their signage.*

GET SMART ABOUT READING LABELS AND LISTENING TO ADS

Some labels can be useful. You're likely to find value-added products like chutney or jam bragging about their local ingredients, cheeses with the farm name right on the packages, and baked goods sold by people who know what they're made of. But smart consumers go beyond the label to read the ingredient list, always remembering that ingredients are listed in order of volume and that the first ingredient makes up the highest percentage of the content.

Remember that labels and ads are often marketing ploys rather than a real effort to give consumers information. Heinz Farmers' Market soup invited consumers to "taste the countryside," implying their vegetables were purchased from the countryside in *this* country when they were actually purchased abroad. I'm sure you're too smart to fall for that, but bear in mind that labels and ads are designed to appeal to your heart. Use your head instead.

And remember that *"organic" does not mean "local."* This isn't a value judgment, just the truth! (See Local vs. Organic on page 13.)

DON'T MAKE ASSUMPTIONS ABOUT FRESHNESS

Is local food always fresher? When you buy directly from the farmer, your food is generally as fresh as it gets. Buying indirectly from retail stores may be convenient, but it doesn't assure you of freshness. I've seen regional apples that were slightly shriveled and unrefrigerated, sitting by the register in a Manhattan supermarket. But, I've also spotted local organic strawberries that perfumed my local co-op with their just-picked smell.

So, once again, go beyond the obvious and use your judgment. If you're in doubt, find out what day the item in question is generally delivered and use the look, smell, and feel of comparable farmers' market or garden foods as a barometer for freshness. Bear in mind that farm-fresh produce may not look as perfect as mass-produced ingredients — especially if it's grown without pesticides or is an heirloom variety — but it should look fresh and not heavily bruised, droopy, or brown. Any produce with cut ends, such as artichoke stems, should look reasonably clean and fresh.

BEWARE OF FARM CHARM

Recently, my supermarket promoted local produce. I really appreciated their attempt and bought some local corn after the manager proudly told me where it came from. But that same day I was also taken in by a charming neighboring display of sweetly packaged "farm items" from the Midwest. (The tiny print at the back of the jars told me the origin of the food.) I have no problem with the jarred goodies from the Midwest. Even better, though, would have been some value-added goods from where I live.

LESS CENTRALIZED = MORE LOCAL

Big box stores and supermarket chains tend to use a centralized distribution system, which discourages local farmers. Happily this method is changing, and so there are exceptions, but generally, the less centralized the buying (as you'll find at independently owned stores), the more likely you will be to find local foods. Small is beautiful. It supports your local economy, too.

THE TIMES THEY ARE A-CHANGIN'

You can change a store's buying policies, or at least get buyers to purchase a specific food from local sources by asking directly, calling, or writing the decision makers. Keep at it, work with local food advocacy groups if you can, and encourage your friends to do the same.

Shopping by Venue

You'll find no permanent rules about shopping for local food in stores because the market is changing continuously, but these tips will give you some general guidelines and a little context when you shop.

SUPERMARKETS

Local food is generally not the focus for most large chain supermarkets, so you have to forage through as many as 40,000 displayed items to find it, if it's even in stock. Their distribution system makes it difficult for local farmers who have to travel far and may be too small to meet minimum quantities.

But there is hope. Some supermarket chains allow discretionary regional buying. Others have someone in corporate headquarters who is sympathetic to the cause of local food or at least is willing to become more educated about it. It's well worth making calls to a company's public relations department and to the food buyers to register your request for more local food. One way to frame your request is to say, "Your competitor, ________, is selling local apples and cider, but you don't. So, even though I'm a longtime customer of yours, I'm shopping there. Is there any way to correct that oversight?"

Some supermarkets, particularly small chains, do make the effort and even feature local foods with targeted promotions, but often only after tremendous pressure from the community. My local supermarket hosted a weekend-long farm stand featuring the local producers that are the store's purveyors.

BIG BOX STORES

Like supermarkets on hormones, big box stores such as Wal-Mart generally have an even more centralized delivery system than regular supermarkets. Although this system can further discourage local buying, some big box stores are making a huge effort to change. It's your job to steer them

Freedom of Choice, but Take My Advice . . .

"At the supermarket you exercise freedom of choice and personal responsibility every time you put an item in your shopping cart, but massive efforts have gone into making it more convenient and desirable for you to choose some products rather than others."

MARION NESTLE
Author of *What to Eat*

> Both increased consumer demand and the rising cost of gas force chains that feature foods from around the globe to reconsider their distribution system and focus more on local foods.

right. Make sure to include requests for food from farms that are sustainable *and* local, as big stores tend to use big farms that may be less likely to use eco-friendly practices. If the big box store near you is doing the right thing, praise them by letter or phone to demonstrate consumer interest and demand. If no local foods are available, contact the store and ask them why. And as always, read labels and signage. Think!

"NATURAL" SUPERMARKETS

While large, natural-food supermarkets like Whole Foods make an effort to buy and promote more local foods than the average supermarket, they still stock more products that are agribusiness organic than those from local, sustainable farms. Be a smart shopper, read labels carefully, and ask when in doubt. Your requests are noticed.

FOOD CO-OPS

Food co-ops, markets that are owned by community members, can be a reliable source for local foods. Many grew out of natural-food buying clubs that put member and community well-being above profit motive. For some, that makes local buying a high priority, and many co-ops are strongly committed to local foods. (In 2008, members of the National Cooperative Grocers Association issued a nationwide challenge called Eat Local America, which invited consumers to increase their local eating to 80 percent during specific dates throughout the summer months.)

But, traditionally, co-op members are focused on organic foods, no matter where they come from. So it is up to co-op members and their boards to push for member education on the benefits of local and sustainably raised foods, which may not be labeled organic (see page 13). Organic food from far away isn't as fresh, leaves a larger carbon footprint, and may come from a large agribusiness organic farm with practices that members don't condone.

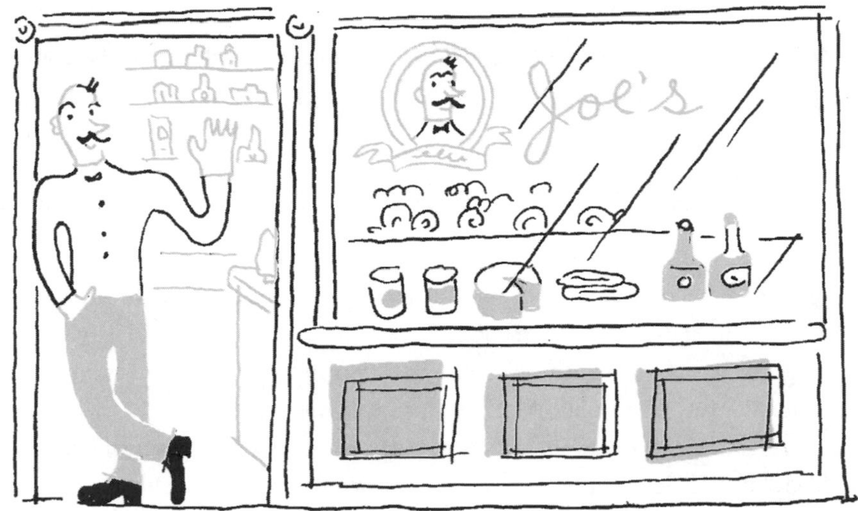

If you're a co-op member, find out what kinds of local food policies are in place. Do they show a commitment to local food? If not, change them!

INDEPENDENTLY OWNED STORES OF ALL KINDS

I've gone from large to small, leaving the best for last. When the owner or buyer is on-board, independently owned stores are the easiest way to find local food. They emphasize customer service, which is in any locavore's favor, and they have the added attraction of boosting your local economy.

Independent stores differentiate themselves from large chains by offering more individualized selections, and they're often more motivated to sell quality products that are produced close to home. If they don't know much about local foods, they may be open to something you bring in. They're less likely to require huge minimum deliveries, so they are a good match for small farmers and food producers who may prefer not to sell to supermarkets anyway.

Single-ingredient stores, such as cheese- or fishmongers, butchers, and wine or liquor stores, as well as health, specialty, and gourmet food shops are generally owned by knowledgeable or at least educable buyers. And of course, individual wineries often have retail outlets.

All-purpose, independently owned mom-and-pop stores still exist, although they're a dying breed. Get to know these store owners; they may be particularly

Keep Trying

When I visited my sister in New York City, I found no local milk at the convenience store next door but four varieties of regional milk in the large specialty store three blocks away.

responsive to consumer requests. Some are solely focused on food; others may sell just a few food items. My local bookstore and the gas station both sell eggs from a local farm. The Public Market, a tiny food market in my town of West Stockbridge, sells local blueberries by the register. I noticed that my local liquor store owner, Ed Domaney, stocks Monterey chevre, a fresh goat cheese from nearby Rawson Brook Farm. That led me to sniff around and notice the large selection of local and regional wines and ciders. When I engaged him in conversation, he told me he went so far as to stock locally made crackers to go with the cheese!

Retail Shopping by Ingredient

Here are some brief tips for buying store-bought local foods.

BEVERAGES

Labeling is usually clear on common local beverages, such water, milk, juice, cider, wine, and other alcoholic drinks. Give preference to those that contain local products and are also processed locally.

Sometimes finding them takes a little work. At the height of the cider season in New England, my local supermarket stocks cider from who-knows-where. But the upscale gourmet food store and local food co-op carry local cider.

Large beverage companies push retailers to buy their line, so keep requesting local products. (For more information about beverages, see page 166.)

DAIRY AND EGGS

Milk is the most common local dairy product available in retail stores large and small. Over the last several decades, all dairies have been hard hit

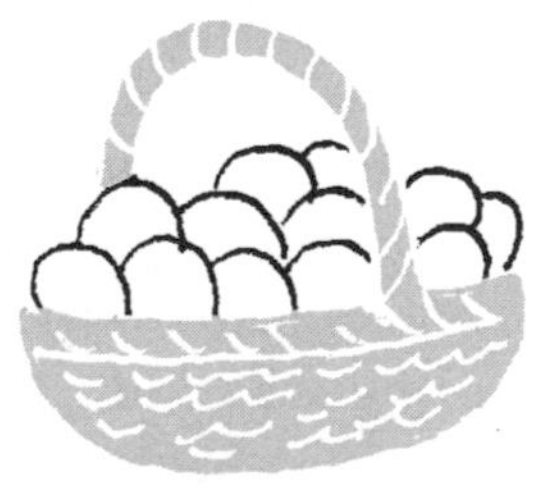

economically, but we are now seeing a resurgence of regional dairies that sell milk to stores. Look for a farm name and location on the carton.

Distinctive local cheeses, many made with local milk, have made a comeback over the last few decades. You may know your local cheeses already from your forays to the farmers' market. If not, a cheese shop, gourmet grocery, co-op, or health food store near you should know what's produced locally. If necessary, call the producer and ask where they sell. Local cheeses from small producers are often not available in supermarkets.

Egg cartons will usually have the farm name right on them, but if you don't recognize it, ask if it is local. As ever, smaller retail stores are more likely to carry them. They can also be found in unexpected places. (What constitutes a sustainably raised egg? See page 167.)

FISH

Wherever you shop, get to know what kinds of fish and seafood are available seasonally from your local fishmonger. If you live near either ocean or the Gulf, you're more likely to find regional fish and seafood than meat and poultry in conventional stores. Nonprocessed fish has to be labeled with its country of origin, but that doesn't take you close enough to the source. So ask.

You may find some surprises, too. My inland supermarket in Massachusetts gets sweet little Maine shrimp in midwinter. But not all the surprises are pleasant. Obvious items like "local" fish may be shipped from elsewhere so local retailers can keep up with the demand. So don't make assumptions.

LOCAL SWEETENERS

Regional sweeteners, including brown rice syrup, sorghum molasses, honey, and maple syrup, are abundant. Even sugar is local in some places. But unless you live near a major producer, you'll need to search small independent stores and food co-ops — or even the farm — to find them. I live in maple country, but I still have to go directly to the farm to buy my honey and maple syrup. Stevia, a plant with extremely sweet leaves, is often sold as a tincture or powder and is most easily found in health food stores. Check the label to see where it comes from, as it is often cultivated outside the country.

If regional seafood is hard to come by, a store in your area might be willing to start a service or buying club for those in search of local fish. (For information about buying sustainable fish, see page 168.)

MEAT AND POULTRY

If no one at the store knows where the meat comes from, it probably isn't local. When it's labeled from a farm or ranch — as it sometimes is in food co-ops, butcher shops, and specialty stores — ask where the farm is. If it's from across the country, ask if there are any closer farms they might buy from. It is painfully hard to find local or even regional meat in mainstream stopping venues today, but we're all working for a change. When you see it, applaud it. (For more about sustainably raised meat and poultry, see page 170.)

PRODUCE

The bottom line? If produce isn't in season in your region and you see it in a retail store near you (see page 17), it isn't local. If it's in season, then it's time to dig deeper and start asking questions. If you're not sure what's in season, print out a regional chart. What's an easy local produce find? In my market, and maybe in yours, it's a paper bag with handles filled with local apples and boldly labeled with the farm name.

VALUE-ADDED FARM PRODUCTS

By adding value to a farm ingredient through any process — such as peeling butternut squash or boiling maple sap for syrup — it becomes a value-added product. The list of these is too broad and variable to cover completely, but it includes baked goods, dairy products (ice cream and yogurt), preserves (salsas, jams, and chutneys), and of course, wine and alcohol.

Snoop around and you'll discover unexpected value-added products, too: pizza made by a local bread company using fresh local basil and goat cheese, apple pie using local McIntosh apples sold at a specialty shop, berry jam made by a neighbor and sold at a convenience store.

The ingredients may or may not originate where these foods are processed. For example, "local" jam in New England may use California

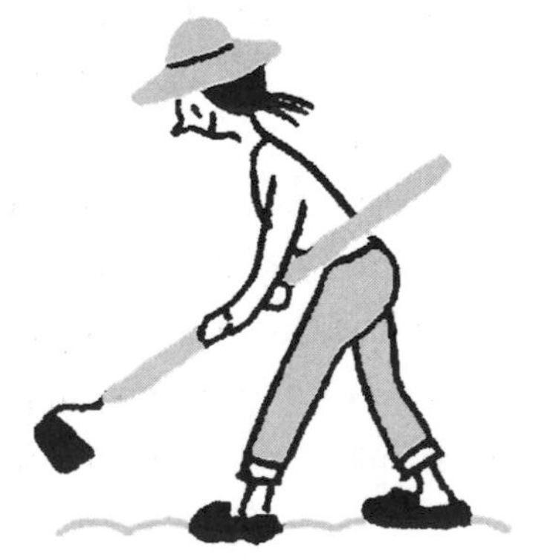

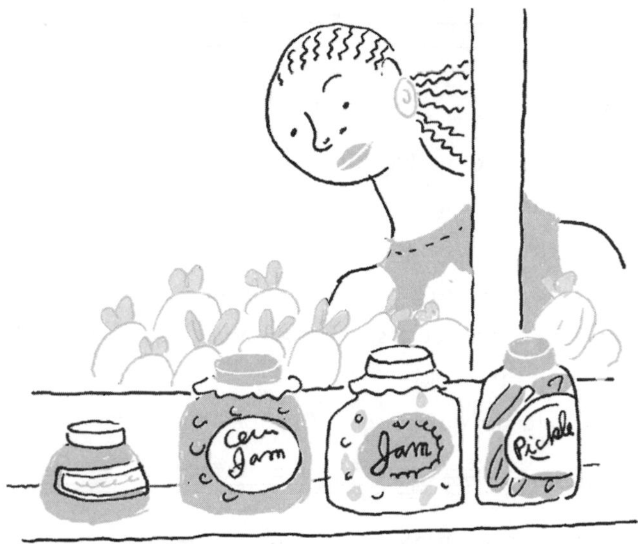

berries that are processed locally. Ideally, *local* means that the ingredients come from your area, but second best is something processed near you — at least it supports local businesses. If you're uncertain, contact the company and find out. (And while you're at it, ask them why they don't use local products, especially if their labeling is misleading.)

Nonperishable value-added products may be proudly displayed. Or they might be out of sight for variety of reasons, including the slotting fees paid by large corporations to place their products in the most eye-catching locations. So hunt. Perishable products tend to be easier to find. Independently owned small stores are more likely to stock perishable and nonperishable value-added products, but pressure is forcing even large venues to make an attempt.

Local Food Not from the Farm

Although the focus of this book is on farm foods, I'm gung-ho on quality foods from local producers, such as local bakeries or coffee roasters who use fair trade coffees. The foods themselves may not be local, but if they are tasty and support business in your neck of the woods, they help build your local economy and create an alternative to large corporate food companies. They're also feeding friends and neighbors, so tend to be more consumer friendly than "big food" is.

Holiday Gift Boxes Done Locally

I taught Tracy how to integrate healthy food into her family's diet. But she taught me how to regain a sense of adventure about local foods through her imaginative gift giving. During the holiday season, way past our growing season, Tracy and her kids still managed to come up with gift boxes featuring a variety of local food items, many purchased at retail outlets. So, instead of generic gifting, she was able to give something with *terroir*, a taste of place. I've added some alternative suggestions, but try creating your own gifts this holiday season and take the journey yourself.

TRACY'S HOLIDAY GIFT BOX

- **Pretty cloth-covered box to hold the gifts.** Tracy used a recycled box she found at a craft store.

- **Red Lion Inn salad dressing.** Locally produced salad dressings are readily available. Or you could make your own using local herbs, maple syrup, olive oil, and citrus. During the growing season, why not add mesclun from the farmers' market?

- **Berkshire Mountain Bakery toasts.** If you can't find toasts, look for locally produced crackers or bread made with local grain, if possible. Other local ingredients include cheese or rosemary. Why not include some jam made from local berries?

- **Monterey chèvre.** Tracy bought fresh goat cheese, produced by Rawson Brook Farm. Include a local cheese from your neck of the woods. And why not throw in a few orchard apples or pears with the cheese? (Remember to deliver your gift quickly if it contains perishables.)

- **Berkshire Brewery Yule Fuel.** This beer is from a local microbrewery. Is there a beverage that's made from ingredients grown near you? Apple or sparkling cider? Wine?

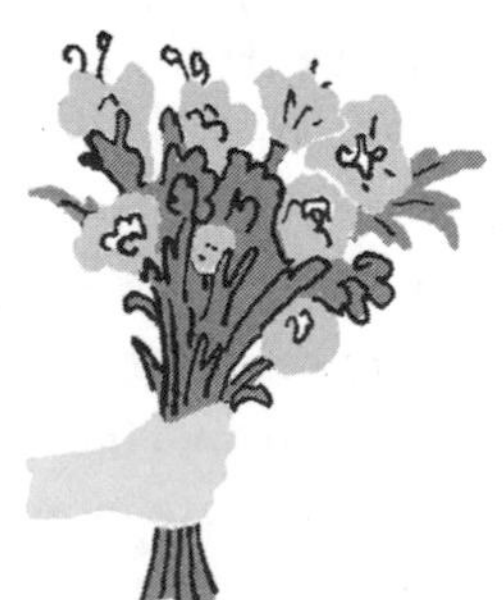

- **Arnoldo's salami.** A local fixture, this old Italian man has been making quality salami for years. Maybe you have an artisan food producer near you?

- **Maple syrup.** If local syrup is not available, give honey. Or make your own pancake mix or muffin mix with local grains. When in season, throw in a box of local berries or fruit to add to the mix.

- **Sweet William ginger cookies.** Who doesn't like cookies? Tracy bought locally made cookies, though you could easily make your own using local butter and eggs. Or buy or make any treats that feature local produce, such as chocolate-dipped strawberries.

- **Baldwin's vanilla extract.** The beans may be from afar, but this extract has been distilled in my hometown by a family business for generations. Choose a product that's made near you and keeps a local company in business.

- **Regional farm and food calendar.** Tracy included a calendar from a local farm advocacy group. This calendar lists what's in season and highlights regional farms, but all kinds of agricultural and culinary calendars are available, some picturing colorful heirloom vegetables. Find them at nonprofit local food initiatives, state agriculture departments, garden centers, restaurants, and agricultural education centers. Or if you come up empty, include a local farm stand or pick-your-own map or a seasonal-focused cookbook.

MAKE YOUR OWN (AND NOT ONLY FOR THE HOLIDAYS)

As you poke around for local food in your region, try a variation of Tracy's holiday gift idea to suit your needs and the occasion. You can buy nonperishable items, like wine or hard cider, anytime, and the perishables shortly before gift time. Of course, if the season is right, include fresh produce from a farmers' market, farm stand, or CSA. Items like freshly picked strawberries and local cream make an instant dessert that can't be beat.

STEP TWO

EAT SIMPLY AND SEASONALLY

We've shopped; now let's eat. Start with opening your fridge to salad greens fresh enough to dance into their bowl, pouring today's cream over strawberries so fragrant they barely made it home, or peeling thick winter carrots that stain your hands orange and taste astoundingly like carrots. These aren't the same sad greens, cardboard megaberries, and sawdust carrots you'd find at the supermarket.

This standout food calls for a new way of cooking. Your food stash isn't just stuff anymore. It feels different, whether your counter's overflowing with summer's bounty or you have just one local item — like a jug of maple syrup boiled off in mid-March, calling out, "Pour me over pancakes!"

You'll want to carry this food's story — where and who it came from — into the kitchen, because it conveys more than its flavor. It connects us to each other. Over local food, strangers bond, friends become friendlier, and even enemies loosen up. It connects us to the culinary traditions of our family, our region, and the season, while encouraging us to create new traditions, too.

Aren't many of the best times you can remember ones that involve food? Highlight local food at holiday dinners, birthdays, or any get-together. Create a celebration from the harvest. Churn ice cream with peaches from your neighbor's tree. Go all out with a corn-and-tomato six-course meal. Or don't do much of anything and let the food speak for itself. Share the shock when people taste thick-cut Brandywine tomatoes from Taft Farms or a little Seckel pear from your CSA share with a dollop of soft blue cheese tucked inside.

Cook alone or ensemble, but cook. Local food lends itself to open recipes and improvisations; methods of preparation are not chiseled in stone but a door to fling open. So walk right in and look around. This food is so good it'll almost prepare itself. (And it's wholesome, too.)

If you don't cook or if you just need a break from it, savor local food raw; no need to embellish. Or go out to eat. Dining out will never be the same once you seek out restaurants and unlikely eateries — from diners to hot dog stands — that embrace local foods. Ever taste freshly ground grass-fed burgers at your neighborhood joint? Ravioli made with foraged mushrooms? Spring greens and local cheese?

After all, this food is the best you've ever eaten. You can taste the life in it.

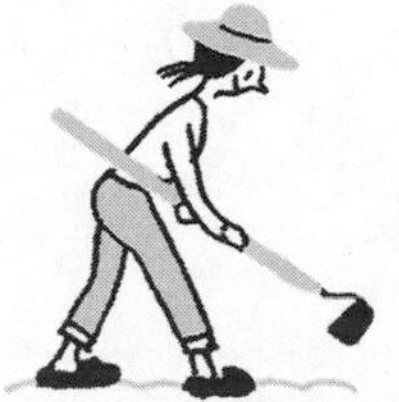

At Home with Local Foods

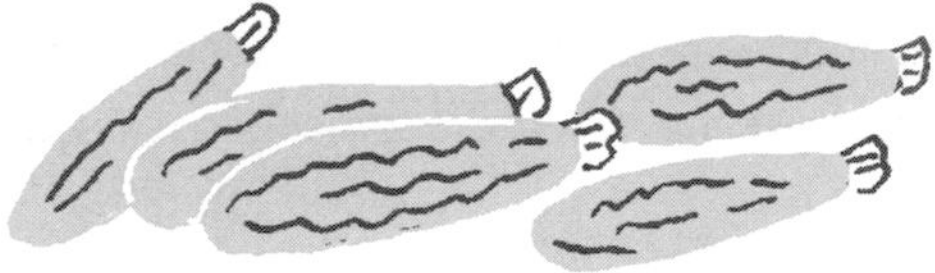

"Make food simple and let things taste of what they are."

CURNONSKY

It's time to get comfortable with local food, integrating it into your lifestyle. Expend as much or little effort as you want, whether you're a skilled cook, queen of the eat-out/take-in set, or someone who falls somewhere in between.

Keep It Simple: Less Is More

If it's fresh and it tastes good, it's gourmet food. Farm-fresh food cooked with minimal ingredients and little skill is often better than food from around the world cooked with dazzling techniques. You don't have to fuss to make it delicious, and often tastier than fine restaurant fare. Cut up crisp apples with fresh local cheese, wok some greens with olive oil and garlic, or top local ice cream with just-picked berries.

Stay Flexible

Don't tie yourself down in the kitchen. You're the boss, so you can set the rules. Don't pen yourself in by consuming a nutritious meal all at once — eat it over a few days if need be. And when time is short, you'll be surprised at what makes a meal: split baked potatoes with local goat cheese warming inside them; a whatever's-in-the-crisper veggie sauté; or pasta with oil and garlic, tossed with a few handfuls of wokked produce. Don't let the concept of the ideal meal stop you from serving a fresh, simply prepared dish for supper.

Share Kitchen Time Together

Most households have a designated cook, but good eating and household relationships get a boost when we all pitch in. If your household has multiple die-hard cooks, actively plan menus and improvise together, switch off cooking nights, or ask everyone to prepare a single dish for a full dinner. If not, move meals along comfortably by sharing kitchen time, not just preparing foods, but also doing the requisite setting and cleaning up. (My marriage vows: I'll cook, you clean.)

Although we've enjoyed glorious cooking times together, especially harvest and holiday meals, neither my husband nor my daughter are enthusiastic about everyday cooking. But, like most households, we've worked out a rhythm. That means they jump in when needed and we're all gratified by the small repertoire of tasty dishes they contribute. Find a local food rhythm that works for you.

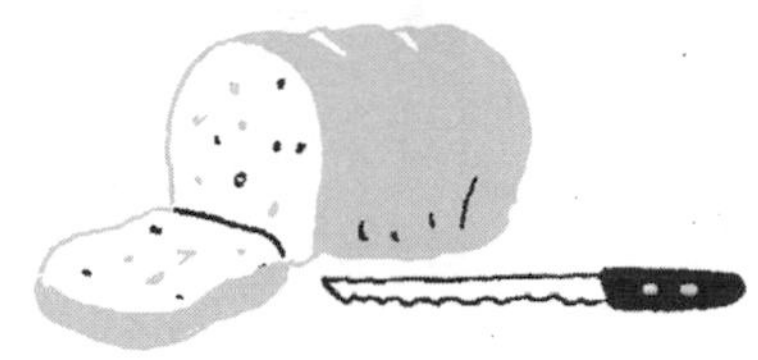

Include Your Kids

Get your kids used to real, unsweetened, unprocessed food as early as possible and do so by example: eat them yourself. That doesn't mean they won't like junk, but at least they'll know the difference.

When you shop, engage your kids in the process, giving them choices whenever possible, seeing that they listen to and relate food-source backstories that you hear along the way. Any chance you get, make trips to direct-from-the-farm venues, like pick-your-own farms, farm stands, and CSAs. Your kids will never forget them.

Cook together, and give kids choices about what to prepare. Those who have a stake in their food are more likely to eat it. Employ them in kitchen tasks, however simple, right from the beginning. The closer they get to the food, the more likely they are to enjoy it, whether it's scraping carrots, snapping beans, or learning to make scrambled eggs. Make homemade versions of kid favorites using local foods. Compare and taste test produce varieties or food sourced from different places, welcoming their feedback.

Introduce new foods as an adventure, with the whole family trying them together. Don't prepare separate meals for fussy eaters, but pull out

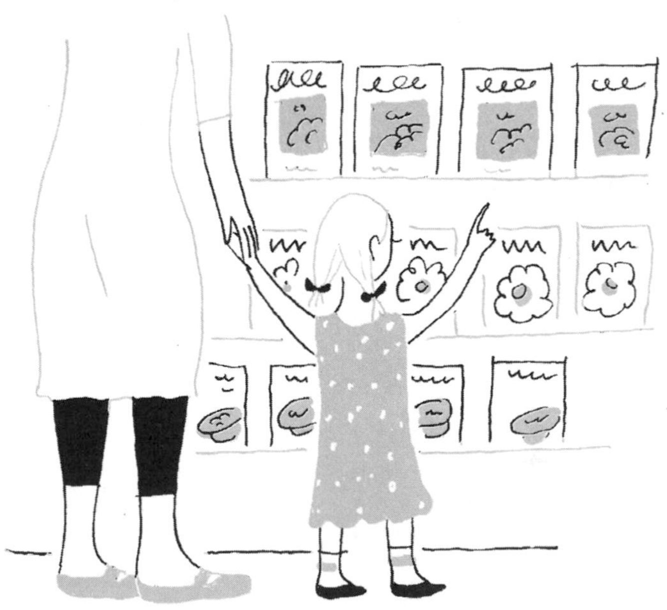

components of your adult meal, separated on the plate, rather than serving them mixed. Or omit the hot spices or eccentric ingredients in the kids' portions. Engage them in foods they like or may grow to like with annual culinary feasts and rituals based on seasonal finds, like shortcake for the first crop of strawberries. (See page 127.) Don't push too hard or make too big of a deal about food, but don't give up either. They may come around later.

Keep Meals Simple

A one-pot meal of fresh local food is better than several processed courses. Make it easier on yourself by serving a premade dish on two nights separated by one freshly made, multiple-course dinner. When you can, double the recipe and freeze half. (See freezing on page 104.) Never underestimate the taste of a fresh steamed vegetable tossed in butter, salt, and pepper.

Enjoy Cooking Solo

Cooking can be the most pleasurable part of your day and often the only time when simple hands-on work gives direct appreciation and pleasure. I often enjoy cooking solo, especially to the right music; it's the ultimate "at home with local food" experience for me when I really have the time. But even workday meals can be a true respite if you keep them simple, take your time, and give yourself over to your senses — the smell, feel, look, and taste of the food. Try it.

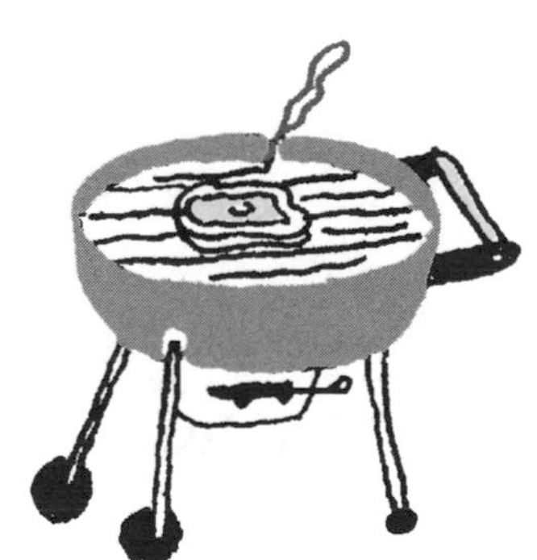

CELEBRATE LOCAL FOOD ON THE HOLIDAYS

Even those who don't cook much may find themselves entertaining (or at least taking a dish to a holiday dinner). You can't ask for a better time to feature local foods and their backstories. Your challenge is to work whatever is local into the meal in the most creative fashion.

EAT YOUR HARVEST

For instant comfort with local food at home, celebrate the harvest of annual crops, such as corn, tomatoes, or strawberries, by preparing and devouring postharvest feasts together.

Think Outside the Box

Try unfamiliar foods as well as heritage varieties of common fruits and vegetables, which will support biodiversity while you munch. As standalone fun or as part of a meal, set up a taste test, casual or formal, to compare and rate varieties of local foods, such as apples, cheeses, tomatoes, or beverages, like wine or cider. Don't label them, so the testers aren't swayed by their prejudices; you may be surprised at the results.

Stock Staple Foods

Local food may be the star, but kitchen staples help it to shine. Setting up your kitchen with pantry and fridge staples empowers you to hang loose and enjoy what's freshest without running around looking for ingredients. I am not a purist, so I use a variety of staples, aiming locally, but ultimately cooking with what brings out the best in local foods, especially during the long winter months in western Massachusetts. Lists of pantry and refrigerator staples abound online. For mine, visit my Web site (see Resources).

Equip Yourself

Although only a knife, cutting board, and a few pots and pans are essential to preparing local food, certain kitchen equipment can help move along your time in the kitchen. If you like tools and enjoy time-saving devices, you'll find lots of fun equipment to help you whip up meals. But don't overbuy. Thousands of unused kitchen tools sit on and under kitchen countertops across America. Bottom line: understand your needs and respect the size of your kitchen. Buy what you think you have room for and will use. For my list of my favorite kitchen essentials, visit my Web site (see Resources).

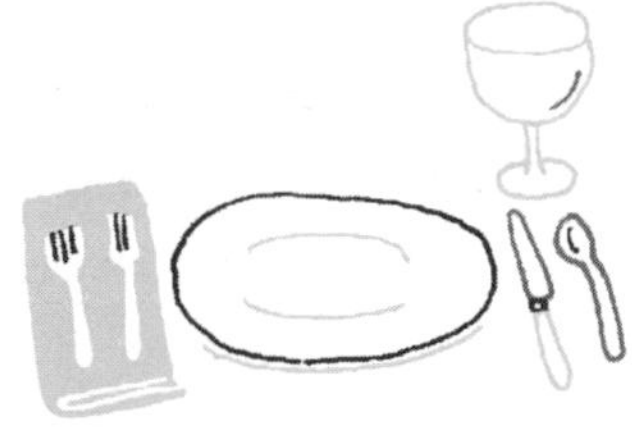

Remember the Seasons

The locavore's kitchen is a seasonal kitchen, ruled by Mother Nature. Getting comfortable with local foods means developing a sense of what's available when. *Once you become familiar with your regional food seasons, everything will begin to fall into place.* Follow your region's local food season once and you'll be on your way, because the rules are generally the same each time. Also follow the link to Sustainable Table (see Resources) to find a guide to seasonal foods in your region; the selections are too varied to include here. Print it out and clip it to the back of this book or keep it in your car for shopping guidance.

Do It Your Way

Anyone who's interested in becoming a locavore must develop a comfort level with local food in his or her own way. Try expanding your local food horizons sustainably rather than seeing the locavore's journey through the classic dieting paradigm of feast or famine, all or nothing. If you're the type of person who likes to plunge in, I applaud you. But you don't have to convert in one short leap. It's fine to buy one or two items to start and move on from there. Sometimes overdoing it can be a turnoff.

There is no single way to include local food naturally in your life. So, I'll guide you sensibly to a comfortable local food life that works with the way you really live. No, I'm not the local food police, checking your fridge for plastic-wrapped iceberg or Argentinian asparagus. So relax and enjoy.

FOR NONCOOKS

If you're intimidated by the thought of cooking or just don't like to cook, you can easily introduce whole local foods, like apples and prewashed mesclun lettuce, into simple meals. And if, like many of us, you dip in and out of cooking, try expanding your repertoire of dishes using the improvisations and open recipes starting on pages 118 and 148. Cooking extends food's lifetime, so turn ingredients into ready-to-eat, healthy meals for later.

FOR INFREQUENT SHOPPERS

Work your fridge, preparing the most fragile-looking (and therefore most perishable) items first. Berries are a good example. Then eat your way toward heartier vegetables, like cabbage, potatoes, and winter squash.

FOR VETERAN COOKS

Those most familiar with cooking often don't use local ingredients, cooking instead from appealing recipes, ideas, or cravings. Stay with that approach, but give it an essential twist: use local, seasonal foods to drive your urges. Design your meals in broad strokes, cooking, as I suggested shopping, for generalized dishes. Cook a seasonal vegetable risotto or soup rather than wedding yourself to specific ingredients with no concern for what's local. That way, you can fill in the ingredients list with what's fresh and ripe. Learn to cook ingredient-focused foods by improvising and substituting. A green is a green; a fruit is a fruit. Making a vegetable tart? Use what's on hand and in season. The results will be considerably tastier and fresher.

Sharing Local Food with Family and Friends

If we don't sit down to savor food with family and friends, what's the point?

Making the effort to build local food into your life gives you time back in a nourished body and soul. You don't have to go anywhere; it's easy to turn a shared meal into something special by setting a delicious tone with good local food and a table lit with candles.

Most people don't entertain all that much anymore, but dining at home is the best way to spend time with friends in a way that's affordable and leisurely. In fact, I enjoy local food most when I'm entertaining, sharing, and savoring my finds with friends. Generally, I host potluck suppers, which are an ideal way to celebrate local food and cut down on cost and preparation while enjoying variety.

But sometimes I fuss and make something sophisticated for the ideal-size dinner party of six, enough company but still cozy. If you go this route, cook plenty of in-season or readily available local food without worrying about repetition of ingredients — it's what's best.

Either way, engage your guests with the story behind the ingredients. For example, the last time you shopped at the Boardman Stand, their rutted road almost turned you back, but the farm's vista makes you feel very *Sound of Music*. Besides, you favor their corn

DINNER PARTY FOR FUN-LOVING ANARCHISTS

If you have a large enough kitchen, ask friends to bring ingredients, unprepped or partially prepared, and cook your dinner together.

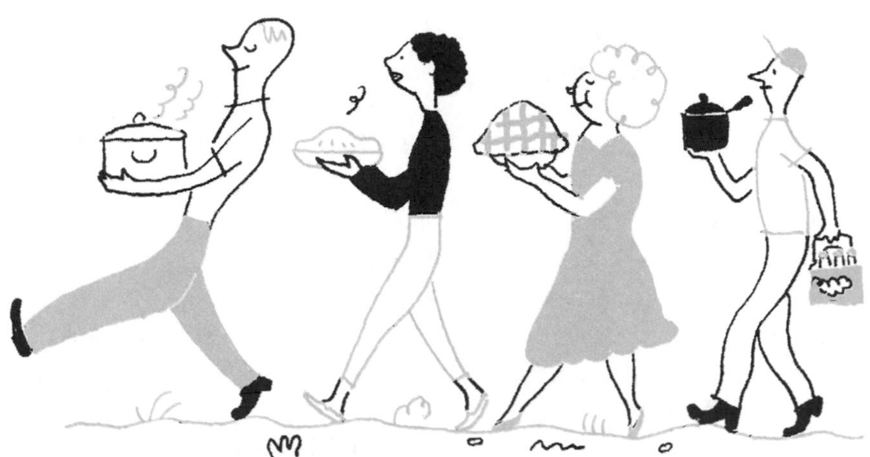

with its less saccharine, much cornier flavor, so you asked the farmer why his corn tastes different. Turns out he doesn't grow the supersweet varieties, designed to produce as much as 10 times the volume of sugar. Then ask your guests, "What do you think of its flavor?"

POTLUCK ENTERTAINING, WITHOUT THE LUCK OR THE POTS

Years ago, after attending a potluck dinner one October night where everyone brought apple pies — 10 pies! — I decided to rein in the luck. It wasn't such a bad party. Once we got over the shock, we all had a laugh and dinner became a pie feast, with diners enjoying slivers of each. But I went home with a bellyache.

Many of the best meals I've had have been at planned potluck gatherings. That may be a contradiction in terms, but the planning cuts down on the time, effort, and cost of entertaining, which can seem daunting especially after a long workweek. Planned potluck entertaining means all you have to do is tidy up and cook one great dish, and you're ready to party. It allows me to easily see people I care about or want to get to know better in a setting where we can enjoy the food and the company.

Generally, I make the main course and everyone brings one dish, not always in a pot. For the most part, my friends are not culinary professionals and some don't even like to cook all that much, but it's easy to make one tasty dish. If not, they can grab a recipe (or a no-recipe idea) from me, from a cookbook, or off the Internet. Those who are too busy, who don't cook, or who I don't know well enough to ask can easily pick up wine, cheese, fruit, bread, dessert, or value-added goodies, such as chutney.

To get started, just send out an e-mail (or call), inviting people to attend. I mention my main dish and give them a choice of what to bring by category, such as appetizer, salad, or dessert. This way I can unleash their creativity (or relax them) without risking redundancy. (Remember those apple pies?) For larger parties, guests are assigned to certain categories. (At one fun wedding I attended, guests were assigned categories based on the first initial of their last name.)

When I'm on comfy turf with friends, I sometimes get more specific and ask them to make something with greens or eggplant or whatever is missing from the mix, or to prepare a dish they've made well before. Parties small enough to sit around the table are organized by course; larger events are set up as a buffet.

You can structure your meal as a bring-your-own-local-food-dish, or if your company isn't already hooked on local food, you could suggest some great sources. You might also give the party a theme, cooking food that emphasizes both the season and your region. During the summer, try a corn and tomato extravaganza; in the fall, host a harvest celebration. Or take your theme out into the world, highlighting cuisine from a specific country or region but still using local ingredients.

Overall, try to keep it simple and fun, and don't ask too much of people.

Prolonging the Seasons 101

Want to save all that great local food for later? Here's a quick overview that covers everything from preserving foods using traditional techniques, as your grandma may have done when she canned her garden tomatoes, to throwing butternut squash soup in the freezer, which I did today. This general course will give you an idea of which methods best suit your lifestyle. Take a look at the excellent books listed in Recommended Reading if you want to learn more.

FREEZING

Freezing isn't the most ecofriendly way to prolong the seasons because it requires long-term use of electricity, but it is one of the tastiest. (I canned things for a few years, then broke down and got a freezer.)

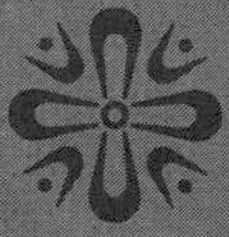

Keeping It Going and Going and Going

"If I have some cherry tomatoes around and I have too much other food that needs to be eaten first, I get out the dehydrator, rinse the tomatoes, slice them in half, and fill up the dehydrator trays with them. In a day or so, I'll fill up a jar or two with these dried gems for winter use. Or if I bought too much sweet corn or the end-of-the-season corn is too tough to eat on the cob, I cut it off and freeze the morsels for winter use. When added to recipes with grass-fed beef, the corn is heaven-sent, even though it would have been starchy and dull if eaten on the cob."

SUSAN SAUTER

Flying Ewe Farm, Treasurer,
West Virginia Farmers' Market Association

Making Stock

Homemade stock is simple to create, and makes use of leftovers that might normally be thrown away. Cover raw or roasted bones, including whole saved poultry carcasses, with water. Add unpeeled onions, celery, and carrots; bring to a boil, skimming the top if you like, and feel free to throw in garlic, herbs, and a splash of local wine. Leave the pot uncovered and simmer, adding water as needed to keep the ingredients covered, for two to four hours or until the stock is tasty with a little salt added. Strain and freeze. (If it's too weak, strain and simmer until it tastes good.)

Don't get too ambitious and freeze more than you can reasonably use in a year. Be sure to date and label everything well. Post an inventory list on the freezer and check off items as you use them. Otherwise you'll have to work your meals around defrosted surprises. (I have, and it's not one of my favorite ways to cook.)

Prepared dishes using local ingredients freeze well, and you'll appreciate them later. So, why not double up on your cooking and freeze the extra? Combined foods, such as soups and stews are ideal, as are herbs and pureed foods. In fact, some gardeners cook their harvested vegetables until soft and puree them to add to soups or serve as-is in the winter. (Try pureed carrot or curried carrot soup!) Some gardeners blanch their overabundance of veggies, one cultivar at a time, in plenty of boiling water, for 1½ to 3 minutes, then cool them immediately in ice water, drain, pack, seal, and freeze. Frozen vegetables are best used in dishes rather than solo; they may retain some of their bright flavor, but their texture changes. I especially enjoy frozen peeled tomatoes (blanch in boiling water then drain and peel) and roasted red peppers.

Fully ripe fruit freezes wonderfully for sauces and cooked dishes. When I'm organized, I go berry picking and freeze blueberries for cooking in pies and muffins and whole strawberries for smoothies. I make applesauce from dropped apples or apple seconds and freeze it. Warm homemade applesauce is a fall tradition in my house; it's a huge kid pleaser, especially if you're used to the jarred yellow stuff. And it's divine in the middle of the winter as-is or with pork.

Frozen sustainably raised local meats and poultry enhance the winter season, too. I buy one-eighth of

How Do I Keep Garlic and Herbs?

Keep whole, uncovered garlic bulbs in a dry, reasonably cool place (but out of the fridge) and away from the light. Chopped garlic can be held in the fridge in oil, or even in sherry or dry vermouth.

Shoppers complain about herbs fading fast, but certain techniques can prolong their usefulness (see pages 129–131). You can dry any herb; rosemary, sage, thyme, and anything in the mint family dry especially well. (For air and salt drying for herb-salt, see page 109 and 110.) Herb plants that go dormant for several months, like rosemary, will stay healthy and productive if given good light and cool temperatures; a sunny windowsill is perfect.

a cow or half of a hog, frozen in cuts for dishes like the Meat-Buying-Club Borscht on page 122. And I squeeze the most out of what can be comparatively pricy meat and poultry by making lots of stock from the bones, freezing it, then using it to cook soups, grains, and sauces. (See Making Stock, opposite.)

Traditional canned condiments like chutneys and jams of any kind also freeze well. Follow recipes, adapting them to local foods if needed, or make up your own. Chutneys require vinegar and a sweetener (if the fruit isn't very sweet), such as sugar or local honey, and a few spices. Jams can be frozen, too; they have a fresher flavor and require much less cooking and sweetener than canned varieties do, especially if you don't require them to be super thick.

If pushed by necessity, you can even freeze cheese (if it's well sealed). Of course, don't forget to freeze baked goods using local ingredients, like some of that homemade applesauce and your neighbor's eggs.

ROOT CELLARING

Live in a seasonal climate? Root cellaring is a traditional storage technique used to hold produce and other foods, such as nuts, seeds, and grains over the dormant season, allowing you to enjoy them throughout the winter when local food is harder to come by.

Start with quality food — mature, unwashed, and unbruised vegetables and fruits. Pack root veggies in sand or sawdust that's damp but not soggy, and store other items in crates or baskets on shelves or at least several inches above the floor for good air circulation. Each

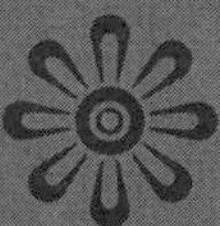

Winter Eats

"The more you can extend your season, the better you'll be eating, and the more you can save. Even without having perfect conditions for vegetable and fruit storage, you can still manage to keep more good food by creative use of odd corners of your house or outbuildings . . . for example, storing squash under the bed in an unheated spare room or keeping apples in an ice chest on an enclosed porch."

NANCY BUBEL

Author of *Root Cellaring: Natural Cold Storage of Fruits and Vegetables*

"Unless I get them at a restaurant, I don't eat greens from California in the winter, as we try to eat locally. My garden cabbages and carrots (50 to 100 pounds of each) as well as potatoes, onions, garlic, beets, apples, etc. get stored in the cold cellar and keep until spring. This May, I still have some cold cellar cabbage I salvaged from last year's harvest in the refrigerator. Our winter salad is shredded carrots and red cabbage, with some feta cheese on top."

JOHN OLANDER

Home gardener, West Stockbridge, Massachusetts

WINTER CSAs

If you want to try the food storage and preservation tips here but don't garden or are unlikely to pick up foods from your local farm stand or farmers' market, consider buying a winter CSA share — the best of winter crops, such as potatoes, carrots, and winter squashes. (To find a CSA near you, follow the link to the Robyn Van En Center in Resources.)

kind of stored food requires a cool place with the right combination of temperature, humidity, and ventilation. (Most vegetables need some moisture, but some, like onions and garlic, like a dry home. Winter squash likes conditions that are on the dry side.)

You'll need to adapt your root cellar to your living conditions, but it can be created indoors or out in a new or preexisting space. Use your attic, the space under your stairs or porch (try packing veggies into foam ice chests), a cool closet, or your garage. Climate permitting, you can even use an unheated outbuilding or room. You can dig an underground root cellar, using buried barrels, boxes, and even a simple earth pit. And sometimes root vegetables can be stored right in the garden, although you'll have to wait until the spring ground thaws to harvest them. (Oh, those sweet parsnips!)

Although some people build elaborate basement root cellars, a basic root cellar simply consists of shelves in a cool, humid basement that has good ventilation. You can also partition a part of the north-facing wall, including a window or installed vent, if possible. If your basement is warm, you'll need to insulate the wall facing the furnace. For additional moisture, if needed, cover the floor with sawdust or sand, sprinkled with water, or keep pans of water near the vent.

For an excellent resource with extensive details, including root cellaring in the city and suburbs, the best cultivars to grow for storage, and much more, read *Root Cellaring: Natural Cold Storage of Fruits and Vegetables* by Nancy Bubel.

DRYING

Unless you live in a very dry climate (think New Mexico), the easiest ingredient to dry simply and naturally is herbs. Buy or harvest some of your own, tie them in bundles with kitchen twine, and hang them upside-down away from moisture and out of direct sunlight. When they're dry and crumbly, slide your hand down the stems in a stripping motion, removing the leaves and sealing them in airtight containers. Some herbs respond well to drying, holding their flavor well, but fragile herbs like basil and cilantro don't. So, I like drying hearty herbs like rosemary, thyme, sage, and various kinds of mint (for cooking and tea). Stevia can also be grown and dried for use as a natural sweetener.

To dry herbs, you can use the sun (best in dry climates), the oven, or the easiest approach, an electric dehydrator. For oven drying, use baking sheets or stretch cheesecloth across your oven racks to create frames. Set your oven as low as possible, 80 to 120 degrees — or, if you have a gas oven, use just the pilot light — and leave your door ajar. Dehydrators come with directions and work well for an overflow of crop or food bought in bulk, from cherry tomatoes to apples, both delicious when dried. Dried fruit, beef jerky, and fruit leather are particularly popular, but dehydrator fans also enjoy dried vegetables. Kathy

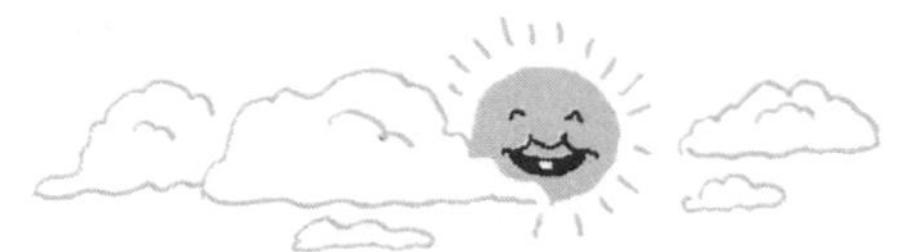

Harrison, author of *Just In Case: How to Be Self-Sufficient When the Unexpected Happens*, dries all kinds of vegetables, especially peppers, mushrooms, string beans, carrots, and onions for thick soups and stews. She also grinds her own dried vegetable combo in a food processor for homemade vegetable bouillon.

Many garden plants can be dried before they're even harvested. Weather permitting, you can dry beans right in the garden on their vines; just leave them in their pods until they rattle. When pods are very dry and shriveled, pick the beans and shell them (fun for kids and adults). Or harvest a bit early and complete the drying process in the sun, an oven, or a dehydrator.

THE MEMORY OF SUMMER LINGERING IN YOUR SALT

About 10 years ago, I started storing rosemary and sage separately in salt. Just break the branches up, or if you prefer, remove the leaves from their stems, and cover completely in kosher salt in a glass jar. The salt will draw out the moisture, so you can use the herb — or, better yet, the herb-salt — for seasoning everything from roasted winter vegetables to chicken.

FERMENTING AND PICKLING

Enjoy beer or sourdough bread? Both of these are examples of fermentation, an age-old way to preserve food by chemically changing ingredients over time. Fermentation is responsible for turning grapes into wine, cabbage into sauerkraut, milk into yogurt or cheese. You can keep these live culture–fermented foods in a cold spot (see Root Cellaring on page 107) or refrigerate them. Pickles can be fermented as well, although quick-pack pickles are simply brined.

Traditional fermented foods are favorites of those who support the preservation of traditional foodways. On the health front, they can also make hard-to-digest ingredients easier to handle, delivering more accessible nutrition.

It's fun to experiment with fermentation, another culinary miracle that allows you to hold excess harvest during the winter months. Fermenting foods is a great local food project to do with the family; it embraces history, food culture, science, and great flavor. For good reading on fermentation, see *Wild Fermentation* by Sandor Ellix Katz.

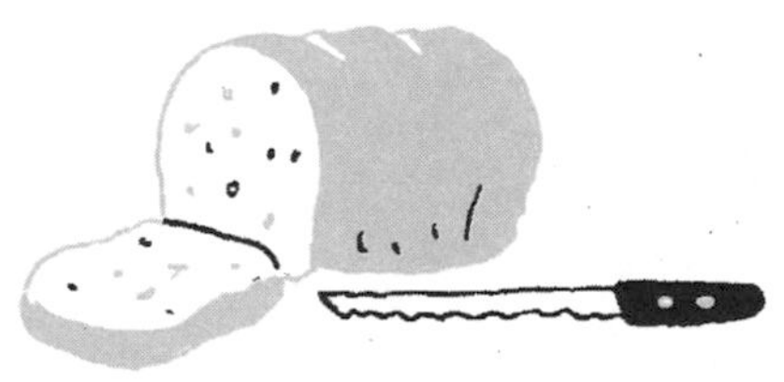

CANNING

Canning seems to be coming back into fashion, especially for those with a little time who don't have the freezer space or who prefer electricity-free storage. Canned harvest treats can be soul-satisfying once it's cold outside and local foods are harder to find. They also make distinctive gifts for the holidays, housewarming parties, and dinner parties.

My advice is not to can everything but to focus on food that tastes great canned. (Some don't. I'm not wild about straight canned vegetables, for example.) But fresh local tomatoes, flavorful pickles, and combination foods, such as homemade ketchups, chutneys, and jams, are especially tasty. Or try whole pears and peach halves in a little brandy. Once you get comfortable with the process, you can begin to experiment if you stay within the timing guidelines and use the proper method.

Depending on the acidity of the ingredients, there are two ways to can, and neither uses much equipment. The boiling-water-bath technique is used for classically canned, high-acid foods, such as pickles, fruits, and vegetables, with enough vinegar to raise the acidity to a sufficient level for safety. It uses a large, deep kettle and rack for holding the jars in place. (I bought a set cheaply at the local hardware store, but you can use any kettle that fits the rack.) Cans are placed in the rack in boiling water. The combination of heat and acidity kills harmful bacteria. Foods with a pH level that's lower or higher than 4.5 must be processed using a pressure canner. Vegetables must be pressure-canned — except for tomatoes, which are a high-acid fruit. When canning vegetable combos, use the longest processing time indicated in the recipe you're following.

Choose canning jars in your favorite sizes with lids and bands to match. Use small jars for jams and larger ones (preferably wide-mouthed to help you get the food inside easily) for tomatoes. The jars need to be very clean and kept hot until ready to use. You'll also need a funnel, hot pads to set the jars on, oven mitts or a jar lifter, a rubber spatula (to twirl out the air bubbles), and standard preparation tools such as sharp knives and a cutting board.

While safety is paramount with canning, it is not difficult to safely can foods if you follow basic rules to prevent bacteria that can cause botulism. Most canning books use USDA guidelines for processing times and proper sterilization of jars. You can double check the USDA 1994 canning guidelines for safety, available online (see Resources for a link).

MAKING YOGURT AND CHEESE

Making yogurt and cheese are age-old techniques that prolong the life of milk. They're well worth trying, especially if you have a connection for high quality fresh milk. While making outstanding artisan cheese is an art form, easy recipes abound for fresh, delicious yogurt, mozzarella, and ricotta. If you want to learn more, read *Home Cheese Making* by Ricki Carroll. She also gives superb classes.

RESOURCES

For good resources and information on prolonging the season, check out the books listed in Recommended Reading.

Open Recipes and Improvisations

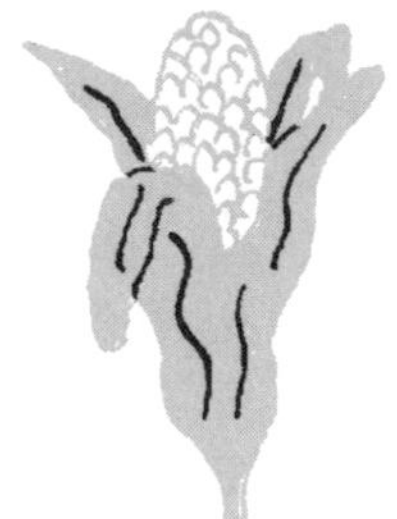

"Sex is good, but not as good as fresh, sweet corn."

GARRISON KEILLOR

Eye-opening flavor was my entry point to the local food journey, and it may be yours, too. Here, we'll savor local food's knack for giving us pleasure by preparing it simply with improvisations and open recipes. (For produce improvisations by ingredient, see page 148.)

Cooking Without Recipes

My cooking students fall into two categories — improvisers and recipe followers. Often, they're married to each other. While recipes can be a boon, especially when you learn to be flexible about adapting them to the local bounty, local food lends itself perfectly to improvisation, which allows you to cook what's in season rather than what's on a list. Besides, it's fun.

IT'S A NATURAL: LOCAL FOOD PREPARATION 101

The truth is that once you've brought local food into your kitchen, most of the basic preparation rules apply, just as they would to any ingredients. The only difference is that you have better materials and thus better results. While a few exceptions to this rule can be found — some produce might need better washing or trimming or may be irregular in shape, and grass-fed meat may require slower cooking — none will break your stride. And for those used to semiprepared foods, such as shucked corn or peeled butternut squash, whole food preparation teaches us how food exists in nature.

The key difference is that freshness and flavor often guide you to do less fussing. Cooking local food is more about paying attention to seasonality and availability than about specialized food preparation.

None of this can begin until you develop a comfortable shop-and-cook rhythm that meshes with your lifestyle.

MORE SAVORING . . .

Continue to savor local food in Play with Your Produce on page 147, a resource jammed with improvisational ideas, all listed by ingredient.

WHEN I SAY "DON'T FUSS," I MEAN IT!

Often the best treat is fresh local produce eaten raw out of hand — an apple, a crisp wedge of fennel, some sugar snap peas, or a juicy peach.

Savor Slow Food

Slow Food is an answer to fast food. It's both an organization and an exciting international movement, which started in Italy and jumped the ocean to the United States. It's composed primarily of decentralized, locally based chapters (called *convivia*), each with its own personality. The convivia celebrate the pleasure of food prepared with regional ingredients shared around a convivial table. If you'd like company-renewing place-based culinary traditions, entertaining with local harvest, sharing recipes, and enjoying regional delights, consider joining or starting a chapter near you. For more about Slow Food and its programs, visit its Web site (see Resources on page 227).

This may take a little practice, so have patience. Pick a few ingredients from your farmers' market on your way home from work. Prepare simple or complex dishes from your twice-a-week shopping, or cook big batches to freeze. Cook for the week on Sundays to the roar of rock music or restrained solo piano pieces. When I'm home in the evenings, I sometimes roast veggies — beets, sweet potatoes, butternut squash, potatoes, or a mix of all of them — to use later when I don't have time. You can also chop vegetables when you do have time, then wok 'em quickly when you don't.

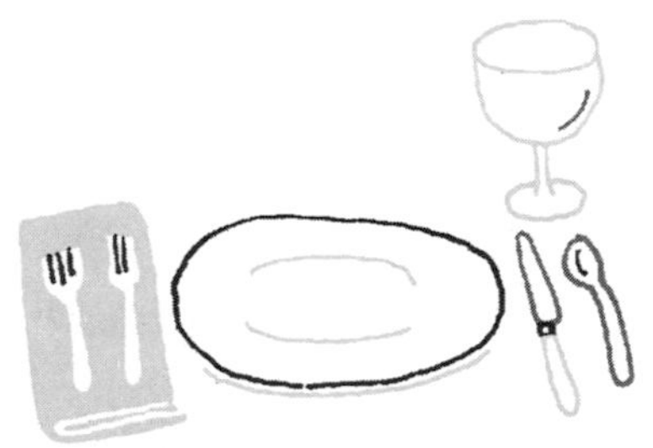

Integrate some kind of local food preparation, however minimal, into the rhythms of your lifestyle, but don't expect to change overnight. The best part? You get to eat the results!

IMPROVISE WITH SIMPLE VEGGIE TECHNIQUES

Play with these structured improvisations using any seasonal produce on hand. (For improvisations by ingredient, see page 148.)

Plunge and Shock (or not)

Plunge vegetable(s) — all cut to the same size — into rapidly boiling, salted water, or steam them in one inch of water using a steamer or covered pot until they are their brightest color. (If you're doing this with a variety of veggies and are including potatoes, cut the potatoes smaller or put them in the water early, as they will need to

NEED A HELPING HAND? TRY AN IMPROVISATION-RECIPE HYBRID

I've included a broad spectrum of improvisational ideas here. Most are fairly simple, but some require more skill. If you're a novice cook but want to try something new, like baking a fresh peach pie, use the suggested improvisation, adapting it to online or cookbook recipes as needed.

cook longer.) Conversely, drop fragile vegetables, such as peas, greens, and mushrooms in the pot immediately before draining.

When vegetables are brightly colored, remove one piece with a slotted spoon to check for doneness. Cook them longer if you like, but they're better undercooked than overdone. Immediately drain the vegetables into a colander when you're satisfied with their doneness — very crisp for dips or additional cooking later, tender-crisp (al dente) for immediate consumption.

Enjoy them right out of the pot, hot and seasoned to taste. Or stop their cooking immediately and keep them crisp by plunging (shocking) them in a bowl of icy water or under a faucet of cold running water until the vegetables are cold to the touch. Use these bright, crisp veggies for salads or dipping, or quickly heat them later in a wok or skillet. To dress, see Plunge and Dress, following.

Plunge and Dress

Follow the directions above. Dress hot or cold vegetables with your favorite dressing, or simply coat them with olive oil and a tiny drizzle of vinegar, or add a squeeze of fresh lemon juice, salt, and pepper. Try Asian flavors, such as soy, freshly grated ginger, and a touch of sesame oil. Or serve them hot with butter, salt, and pepper, or with olive oil that has been simmered briefly with a little garlic.

For effortless pasta dishes, use this technique: Just throw vegetables, such as broccoli florets, into the pasta water during the last few minutes of cooking, then drain them together with the pasta. Dress the dish with garlic simmered in oil or whatever you like. Again, the more fragile veggies, like greens, go in at the very end.

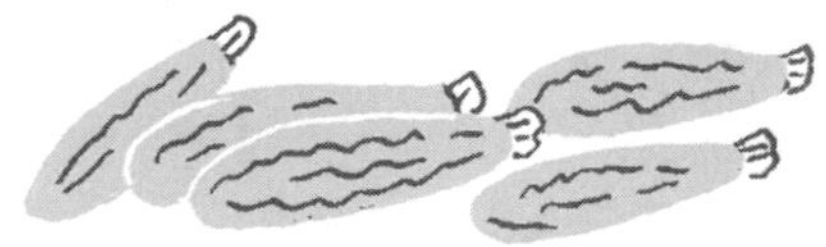

Toss and Roast

Toss vegetables in olive oil to lightly coat (adding minced garlic and/or herbs, if you like), and spread them onto a baking sheet in one layer. Roast at a high heat, 400°F to 425°F, shaking the pan or stirring occasionally to prevent sticking, until browned. This technique works particularly well with root vegetables. See Roasted Harvest Vegetables (page 125) as a model for other vegetables. The method is also a tasty way to prepare individual vegetables, especially asparagus and string beans.

Brush and Grill

Lightly brush or toss vegetables with olive oil (plain or seasoned with garlic and/or herbs). Grill over medium heat, turning once or more as needed, until just tender. Eggplant, thickly sliced onions, whole or halved bell peppers, and whole tomatoes work well this way, but you can experiment with all kinds of fruits and vegetables. Some vegetables, such as asparagus, respond well to quick plunging and shocking first (see Plunge and Shock on page 115).

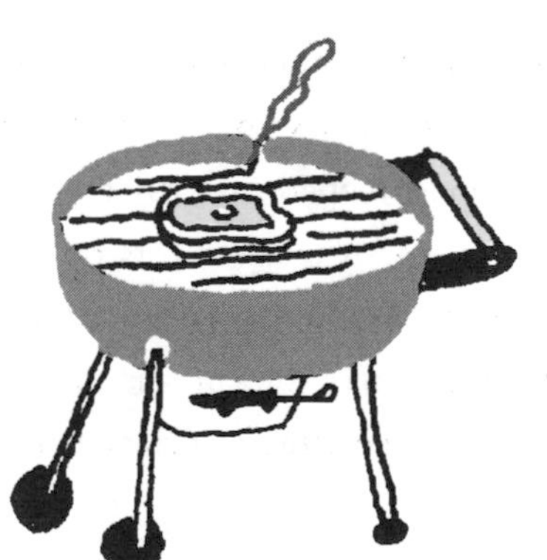

If you're cooking with a charcoal grill, don't waste the heat after you've finished cooking your meal. Cook whole vegetables — such as potatoes, eggplants, and onions — as-is or wrapped in foil in still-hot, but slowly cooling, covered grills.

Soup

Combination vegetable soups are forgiving dishes and thus are ideal for harvest improvisations. For soup, adapt a recipe using what's locally available, or simply simmer vegetables in a flavorful broth and add chopped herbs or cooking greens just before serving. Or for a pureéd soup, simmer root vegetables, such as onions and carrots, in broth with seasonings and garlic until soft, then blend them in a food processor and season to taste. Experiment or adapt recipes to local foods. Of course, meat, fish, or poultry can be added for a flavorful boost (see Meat-Buying-Club Borscht on page 122).

Everything Salad

Get flexible with your salad ingredients. Toss your best local finds with simple dressings (see page 118 for some ideas). Salads may contain greens, vegetables, fruit, or a combination of all.

Try pairing tangy greens, like arugula, with sweet fruit, like oranges. Toss plunged and shocked vegetables (see Plunge and Shock on page 115) into cold cooked pasta, grain, or potato salads. Combine vegetables with cooked meat, fish, or poultry for excellent salads as well. You are limited only by your imagination.

Harvest Vegetable Risotto
In half an hour from beginning to end, you can adapt a plain or vegetable-based risotto recipe by adding local, farm-fresh vegetables cut into small pieces for a meal in one. You don't want the veggies to be crisp, so add them during the beginning or middle of cooking, or even the end if they were roasted or sautéed beforehand. Vegetables that need little time to cook, such as greens, can also be added at the end. If you are using fresh herbs, throw them in at the end, too.

Open Recipes

The following recipes are what I call "open recipes" — they don't require precision and they allow you the flexibility to substitute seasonal local foods. Use them as a model to learn how to adapt your own recipes to what's available near you. Enjoy!

DRESSING YOUR FRESH GREEN SALADS

Always toss a green salad immediately before serving, with just enough dressing to coat; it shouldn't be sopping. The perfect instant dressing can be made at the last minute: simply toss greens lightly in a great-tasting olive oil with a touch of kosher or sea salt. Then toss again with just a touch of vinegar or a squeeze of lemon juice. (Less is more.)

For a classic vinaigrette assembled American-style, pour into a small jar 1 part vinegar to 3 or 4 parts oil, depending on how tangy you like it. Add a touch of Dijon mustard, salt, and, if you like, some chopped shallots or garlic. Shake. (My mom uses a baby bottle so she can measure ingredients on the side.) For an easy Asian-style dressing, try a milder oil and rice vinegar, freshly grated ginger or chopped pickled ginger, a tiny touch of sesame oil, and a pinch of sugar. Dressings can be also made with citrus juice instead of, or combined with, vinegar. Play!

Market Salad with Pan-Roasted Potatoes and Cheese

Opposites attract in this last-minute dinner salad of warm potatoes and cool greens sprinkled with the best local cheese available. (This is a growing- and shoulder-season recipe.)

4 medium red potatoes (or your favorite thin-skinned market potato)

4 tablespoons olive oil

1 large head of your favorite lettuce, or 6 cups of mixed greens

16 cherry tomatoes, halved, or 2 of any kind of tomato, cut into small wedges

4 thin slices of red onion or any sweet onion, separated into rings

3 to 4 ounces of tangy local cheese, crumbled, diced, or grated

Salt, preferably kosher or sea

2 garlic cloves, coarsely chopped

1 tablespoon red wine vinegar

Freshly ground black pepper

Serves 3 to 4

1. Cut each potato into bite-sized pieces. Preheat a large cast-iron skillet or any heavy skillet over medium-high heat for 2 to 3 minutes. Add 2 tablespoons of the oil. (It will start to smoke.) Carefully and quickly place the potatoes in the pan, cut sides down. Sear until nicely brown, 5 to 7 minutes, shaking the pan vigorously or turning the potatoes over with tongs, until fork-tender, another 5 to 7 minutes.

2. While the potatoes are roasting, wash and dry the lettuce. Tear the lettuce into bite-sized pieces and divide them among 3 or 4 plates or shallow bowls. Scatter the tomatoes, onions, and cheese equally over the greens.

3. When the potatoes are fully cooked, salt them generously in the pan, then arrange them over the salads. Let the pan cool off the stove for a minute to prevent burning, then add the garlic. Return the pan to the stove and cook, stirring constantly, just until it starts to brown very lightly. Immediately whisk in the remaining 2 tablespoons of oil and the vinegar. Drizzle the dressing over the salads. Add pepper to taste.

Local food improvisation: Nothing here is chiseled in stone. This salad is served on mild lettuce, but I like it equally well on bitter greens, such as a head of escarole with a bunch of arugula. It's your choice. Feel free to use whatever local cheese is available — I love blue cheese. If you want to use a soft cheese, spread it onto a small piece of toasted bread or baguette slice, but also add a touch more dressing to compensate for the zing of the on-salad cheese. You can also add other seasonal items, such as carrots, peppers, local hard-boiled eggs, leftover roasted chicken, or crispy bacon.

Abundant Harvest Oven-Dried (or Roasted) Tomatoes

If you don't live in a hot, dry climate and don't have a dehydrator to save the season's bounty, oven-dry or roast tomatoes just until their flavors are wonderfully concentrated. (This is a growing-season or end-of-the-harvest recipe.)

5 pounds tomatoes (plums are easiest, but use whatever you have)

Olive oil to coat very lightly

3 minced garlic cloves (optional)

1 tablespoon fresh or 1 teaspoon dried herbs (optional)

Kosher or sea salt

1. Preheat the oven to 200°F.

2. Remove the tomatoes' stems, then cut the tomatoes in half lengthwise. Toss with the oil, garlic, and herbs, if using, and salt to taste. Arrange, cut sides up, in one layer close together but not touching, on baking sheets (preferably parchment-covered or nonstick).

3. Roast until half-dried or dried and shriveled, between 6 and 12 hours. (Taste and remove them anytime you like, but only totally dried tomatoes can be stored at room temperature.) Different sizes of tomatoes will dry at different times, so remove them as they are done if the batch dries unevenly.

Yield varies greatly depending on how long you dry the tomatoes

To store: Store very dry tomatoes in a sealed bag at room temperature. Reconstitute in water, broth, or right in a sauce of any kind. Store roasted (half-dried) tomatoes in oil in the fridge for several weeks or, as I do, as-is in a plastic container in the freezer.

Serving suggestions: Enjoy half-dried (roasted) tomatoes with olive oil (and garlic and herbs, if you like) in an antipasto, over pasta, in any kind of sauce, or puréed with nuts and cheese for a spreadable tomato pesto. They're also great in any kind of sandwich.

Quick roasted sauce variation: Savvy Tammy Jervas, food service director at the tiny school near me in Richmond, Massachusetts, buys end-of-the-season tomato seconds from her local farm. She cores them, removes any blemishes, then roasts them, drizzled with oil and sprinkled with a little sugar, on parchment paper in a 400°F oven. (About 5 pounds of tomatoes will require ¼ cup of oil and 1 tablespoon of sugar.) When they are soft enough to break up, about 45 minutes later, she does just that, then continues to cook them 15 minutes more or until they brown. Then she adds lots of whole peeled garlic cloves and roasts them about 15 minutes more until the cloves are soft. To finish, she blends this ambrosia in a food processor, adding salt to taste and basil, for a fresh and freezable sauce.

Smashed Potatoes and Celery Root with Chives

The combination of potatoes and celery root (a knobby root also called celeriac) is a satisfying culinary classic. If you can't find celery root, feel free to replace it with your favorite root veggies, such as sweet parsnips and/or tangy turnips, along with a couple of peeled garlic cloves — all will yield excellent results. I've used traditional russet potatoes here, but use whatever potatoes you like, leaving the skins on if they are tender. This recipe is adapted from my first book, One-Pot Vegetarian Dishes. *(This is a fall shoulder- or dormant-season recipe.)*

3 pounds baking potatoes (about 6), such as russet, peeled and cut into ⅛-inch pieces

1 small celery root (about 1 pound), peeled well and cut into ½-inch pieces

¼ cup butter, or more, melted

About ½ cup milk, chicken broth, or vegetable broth, or more if needed

Generous amount of salt and freshly ground black pepper

2 tablespoons or more chopped chives, scallion greens, or fresh parsley

Serves about 8

1. Fill a large saucepan with about 1½ inches of water, inserting a steamer if you have one. Add potatoes and celery root. Bring the water to a boil. Cover tightly and cook until the vegetables are soft, about 25 minutes, stirring once.

2. In a large bowl or right in the pot, use a potato masher to smash the potatoes and celery root, adding about 2 tablespoons of the butter and stirring in milk to reach the desired level of moisture. If you don't have a masher, fear not — you can make do with a large spoon or a mixer. Do not use a food processor, however; it will make the vegetables gummy. Season with generous amounts of salt and pepper to taste. Blend until well combined but a little lumpy. (Or if you're a purist, blend until smooth.)

3. Mound the vegetables into a warm serving dish. Drizzle with the remaining butter and sprinkle with chives. Serve immediately.

Local food improvisations: See variations with other root vegetables, above. If you adore the flavor of chives, mix an extra 2 tablespoons into the smash. Or drizzle the finished dish with pretty green chive butter (recipe follows) and chives. If you like garlic, add 5 peeled garlic cloves to the cooking vegetables.

Chive Butter: To make chive butter, blend chives and melted butter in a blender. Strain the mixture through a fine sieve, and drizzle it over vegetables. Sprinkle the dish with reserved chopped chives. (Also try chopped fresh parsley or dill instead of chives.)

Meat-Buying-Club Borscht

This hearty Moscow-style borsht continues to get better over the course of several days and freezes well, so double the recipe. I use any cut of meat I have from my eighth-cow order (except the more tender steaks), sometimes adding the bones for flavor and then removing them at the end of the cooking time. I use a food processor to shred the veggies, radically cutting down on preparation time, but they can be sliced or diced, too. (Best as an end-of-the-tomato-season recipe or dormant-season recipe if you use canned or your own roasted tomatoes. *See page 120.)*

¾ pound beets, tops and most of stems removed

1¼ pounds boneless beef chuck roast (or any stewing meat), cut into bite-sized cubes

Flour

3 tablespoons vegetable oil

1 quart water or beef stock, or some of each

1¼ pounds tomatoes, peeled* and coarsely chopped, or 1 (28-ounce) can diced tomatoes, drained

3½ cups shredded cabbage, any kind

2 carrots, shredded

2 celery ribs, shredded

2 small or 1 large onion, chopped

1. Preheat the oven to 400°F. Wrap the beets in foil, and roast them until they are easily pierced with a fork, about 1 hour. Set the beets aside until they are cool enough to handle.

2. Meanwhile, toss the meat in a bowl with a little flour until lightly coated. Remove the meat, leaving most of the flour behind. In a large pot, brown the meat in one layer in the oil over medium-high heat, shaking the pan and turning the meat as it browns. (Do it in two batches if necessary.) Don't worry if some sticks or if the meat doesn't brown evenly.

3. Add the water and/or broth and tomatoes, and simmer gently until the meat is almost tender, about 1 hour or more. (Taste it!)

4. Add the vegetables and tomato paste. Simmer gently for another 30 minutes or until the meat is very tender. (If necessary, add extra water or stock to reach the texture of a thick soup.)

5. Prepare the roasted beets by removing any remaining stems, slipping off and discarding their skins, and grating them in the food processor. Add the grated beets to the soup.

6. Season with the vinegar, lemon juice, garlic, salt, pepper, and sugar, if using. Simmer for 15 minutes. Serve with sour cream and chopped dill, if using.

1 tablespoon tomato paste

1 to 2 tablespoons red wine vinegar

1½ to 2 tablespoons lemon juice

2 to 3 cloves garlic, minced

Generous salt and freshly ground black pepper

1 tablespoon sugar (optional)

Sour cream, crème fraiche, or yogurt (optional)

Chopped fresh dill (optional)

*Tomatoes are easily peeled by dropping them briefly into boiling water.

Local food improvisation: Use this recipe for any beef stew with seasonal veggies, leaning more to the meat or veggies as you see fit, omitting the beets and the end-of-recipe seasonings, and adding variations such as fresh thyme or rosemary. If you don't have tomatoes on hand, omit them and add a splash of local wine.

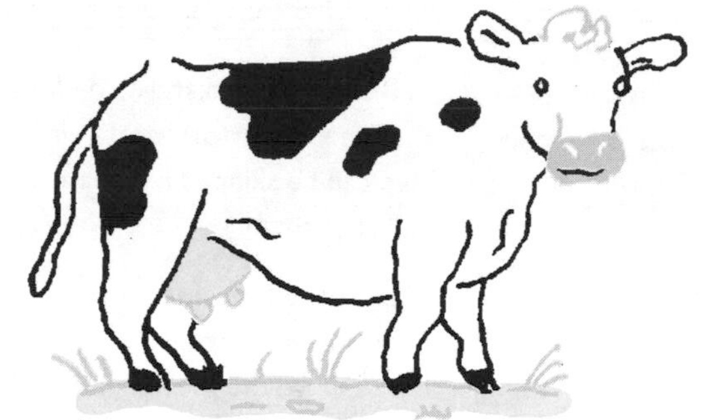

Makes about 2½ quarts. Can be easily doubled or tripled to freeze.

SNACKING ON KALE

For a healthful snack, try crispy kale. Remove tough stems, and tear or chop a bunch of kale. Wash, dry, and toss with just a touch of olive oil and salt (or replace the salt with just a touch of grated hard cheese). Place the kale in a rimmed baking sheet in a preheated 350°F oven; roast, stirring once, until crisp to the touch but still green, about 10 to 12 minutes.

Wokked or Braised CSA Greens

Of course you can buy them anywhere, but CSA farmers frequently tell me that the question most asked by members is, "What do I do with cooking greens?" Here are two answers: braise or wok, both quick methods, which can be used on any greens, wild or cultivated. Braising mellows and softens hearty greens that some folks find too strong or tough, such as kale, collards, turnip greens, or mustard greens. Wokking (or sautéing) works well for more fragile mild greens, such as spinach or chard. (This is a growing- or shoulder-season recipe.)

1 bunch of any kind of cooking greens (see Greens, Cooking on page 157)

2 to 4 tablespoons olive oil

2 garlic cloves, thinly sliced

¼ cup chopped onion or scallion (optional)

Kosher or sea salt

Vinegar or fresh lemon juice (optional)

Serving suggestions: Serve as a side dish, or enjoy for a light dinner with raw sliced red onion, toasted French bread, and local cheese. Toss with pasta solo, or add cooked potatoes and/or crispy bacon.

Makes 2 to 3 servings; easily doubled

1. Remove and discard the long ends and tough spines from the greens. Tear or cut the greens into bite-sized pieces. (This step can be skipped if you are braising.) Some cooks like to roll and slice them.

2. If you're braising. In a medium skillet, heat the oil and garlic until it is fragrant but not brown. Remove the skillet from the heat. Plunge the greens (and onions or scallions, if using) into a large pot of salted, boiling water, and immediately drain them into a colander. (Alternatively, if you like your greens milder, you can cook them for up to 10 minutes.) Press the water out with a spoon. (If you haven't torn or chopped them, you may chop them a few times with a knife, although this step is not essential.) Immediately go to the wok step below or toss the greens with the garlic oil. Season to taste with salt and, if using, vinegar or lemon juice.

If you're wokking or sautéing. In a wok or large sauté pan, heat the oil over medium heat. Add the garlic (and onion or scallion whites, if using). Cook, stirring occasionally, until the garlic is fragrant but not browned and the onion is translucent. Add the greens (and scallion greens, if using), and cook, turning them with tongs, until the greens are warm and wilted, about 2 minutes. Season with salt and, if using, vinegar or lemon juice.

Variations: Drizzle braised greens with a hot vinaigrette or browned butter. Wok greens with tomatoes or bacon. Season wokked greens with an Asian dressing or hot sauce.

Roasted Harvest Vegetables

Use this toss-and-roast method for whatever's on hand, checking for doneness and, if necessary, removing anything that cooks a bit faster. Experiment. I love roasted sweet potato chunks, and kids enjoy cubed butternut squash tossed with butter, maple syrup, and cinnamon. The recipe is from my first book, One-Pot Vegetarian Dishes. *(This is a growing- or shoulder-season recipe. Leave out the peppers for a dormant-season recipe.)*

¾ pound red potatoes, or any potato, cut into 1-inch pieces or wedges

½ large sweet onion, cut into 1½-inch-thick slices

2 bell peppers, any color, cut into eighths

2 carrots, cut diagonally into ½-inch-thick slices

¾ teaspoon fresh rosemary leaves, or ½ teaspoon dried rosemary

1 to 2 garlic cloves, minced

About 1½ tablespoons fruity olive oil, or more to coat very lightly

Kosher salt and freshly ground black pepper

Serves 3 to 4 as a side dish; easily doubled using 2 baking sheets

1. Preheat the oven to 425°F. Toss together everything except the salt and pepper.

2. Spread the vegetables in a single layer on a baking sheet. Roast, turning the vegetables occasionally to prevent sticking, until the potatoes are cooked through and lightly browned, 30 minutes or more. Immediately sprinkle the vegetables with kosher salt and pepper to taste. Serve.

Dan Barber's Pickled Fennel

Almost anything can be pickled, and fabulous pickled cucumber, sauerkraut, and kim chi recipes abound. So here I've given you something different from Dan Barber of the restaurants Blue Hill and Blue Hill at Stone Barns — a simple, tasty refrigerator pickle recipe that uses fennel. (This is a growing- or shoulder-season recipe.)

3 medium or 5 small fennel bulbs

½ teaspoon black peppercorns

½ teaspoon fennel seeds

12 ounces rice wine vinegar

2½ tablespoons sugar

1 tablespoon salt

Thyme sprigs

Makes 1 quart

1. Remove the tops of the fennel bulbs. Peel and discard the outer layer of the bulb if it is tough. Slice the fennel thinly, preferably on a mandoline or hand slicer.

2. Place the peppercorns and fennel seeds in a medium pot; cook, stirring over medium heat until they are lightly toasted.

3. Add vinegar, sugar, and salt; bring to a simmer. Add the sliced fennel.

4. Remove the pot from the heat. Add the mixture to a quart-sized jar with a few thyme sprigs and refrigerate. The pickles are excellent after 12 hours and will be at peak flavor for 2 weeks in the refrigerator.

Serving suggestions: Great with fish, sandwiches, charcuterie, and even in salads.

Pick-Your-Own Strawberry (or Any Berry) Shortcake

After our annual picking at Ioka Valley Farm, our favorite feast is strawberry shortcakes with warm, dense biscuits and fresh whipped cream. I sometimes plan ahead, making biscuits before we pick, then storing them, uncooked, in the freezer on parchment-lined sheet pans. That way, they're ready to pop into the oven for an ideal strawberry shortcake supper on our return. It's our once-a-year dessert-for-dinner meal. (This is a growing-season recipe.)

Berries

3 pints local strawberries (or any local berry)

Sugar

Biscuits and cream

2 cups flour, local if possible

2 to 4 tablespoons sugar

1 tablespoon baking powder

1 teaspoon salt

1⅔ cup heavy local cream

4 to 5 tablespoons local butter, melted

Makes 12 shortcakes, about 6 generous servings

1. Preheat the oven to 325°F.

2. Hull (or cut the tops from) the strawberries; slice. In a medium bowl, mash slightly with a potato masher or large spoon until very coarsely chopped. Stir in sugar to taste and set aside.

3. Sift together in a medium bowl the flour, a heaping tablespoon of the sugar, baking powder, and salt Add 1 cup of the cream, and mix the dough with your hands or a rubber spatula. Knead no more than a minute, just to bring the dough together. Turn the dough onto a lightly floured board or counter. Pat it into a square about ½ inch thick. Cut the dough into 12 squares or use a biscuit cutter to cut 12 rounds.

4. Cover a baking sheet with parchment. Pour half of the melted butter onto the baking sheet. Place the biscuits on top, and pour or brush the remaining butter over each. Bake 12 minutes, or until the tops just begin to brown.

5. While the shortcakes are cooking, with a hand whisk or an electric beater set on high, whip the remaining cream just until it forms soft peaks, seasoning it to taste with a touch of the remaining sugar.

6. Split the biscuits gently by hand or with a fork, and place on 6 plates or in 6 shallow bowls. Top the bottom halves with the berries and whipped cream. Place the second halves on top. Or let diners prepare their own feast. Eat immediately!

U-Pick Best Fruit Kuchen

This tasty confection is a variation on Jane Brody's popular plum tart recipe, published in the New York Times *years ago, and is a very loose adaptation of a German kuchen. It's a snap to make and excellent for a brunch or potluck sweet. (This is a growing-season recipe.)*

1 stick (4 ounces) unsalted butter, softened

1 cup sugar

2 eggs

½ teaspoon almond or vanilla extract

½ teaspoon ground cardamom

1 cup flour

1 teaspoon baking powder

Best of the fruit harvest (see variations below)

Ground cinnamon

Granulated sugar

Squeeze of lemon juice

Confectioners' sugar

1 to 2 tablespoons sliced almonds (optional)

Serves 8

1. Preheat the oven to 350°F.

2. Using a mixer, food processor, or wooden spoon, mix the butter, sugar, eggs, extract, and cardamom until combined. Add the flour and baking powder, and blend again until combined.

3. Generously grease an 8- or 10-inch springform pan. (Or better yet, use a nonstick one.) Add the batter and spread evenly. Lay the fruit on top, close together in a pattern. Dust with cinnamon and a generous amount of sugar; drizzle with the lemon.

4. Bake for 50 minutes to 1 hour, or until well browned on top and sides.

5. Dust with confectioners' sugar. If using, toast almonds in a dry pan over medium heat, stirring. Sprinkle over kuchen. When the kuchen is cool, remove the cake; run a knife along the side of the pan if it sticks.

Local food improvisation

Try these or experiment with whatever's been freshly harvested.

• 2 peeled and sliced apples or pears, lightly tossed in cinnamon and nutmeg or a touch of exotic garam masala. Overlap them slightly in concentric circles.

• 2 cups of blueberries, tossed with a touch of maple syrup and a little flour to coat.

• 12 prune plums, halved lengthwise, pitted, and pressed cut-side down in circles.

Herbs: Open Recipe Extravaganza

What do you do with the rest of your unused bunch of herbs when the harvest is overwhelming or you just want to taste green in the winter? Here are some ideas. The general directions can be used for all herbs unless noted otherwise.

GENERAL PREPARATION DIRECTIONS

Wash and dry the herbs well, but be gentle with their tender leaves so as not to bruise them. The texture of these green concoctions is up to you; they can be smooth or slightly coarse. Chop the herbs by hand, blend them with a food processor, or mash them with a mortar and pestle.

While herbs are best used fresh, they freeze well enough to be a tasty winter surprise. So, for individual servings of the open recipes below, spoon them into ice cube trays. When frozen, pop them out and store them in plastic containers in your freezer. For more information on herbs, see page 107 (general preserving), page 109 (drying), and page 110 (salt preserving).

Although the main local ingredients here are herbs, don't forget to seek out other local goodies — garlic, nuts, and cheese — freely substituting what's available. I'm no fundamentalist, so although it isn't produced near me, I won't give up my olive oil. But if you prefer, use local butter if you are making a warm dish, or combine melted butter and local oil.

EASY HERB PREP

Parsley and cilantro stems, unless very thick and tough, are fine to add to any recipe, especially one that is blended.

Traditional Basil Pesto

Blend until smooth or almost smooth: 3 cups loosely packed basil leaves, 2 chopped garlic cloves, about ½ cup olive oil (or oil and softened butter combined), and 2 heaping tablespoons of nuts (such as pine nuts, walnuts, or pecans). When ready to serve, mix in 2 tablespoons to ¼ cup grated or shredded hard grating or Parmesan cheese. Mix just to combine.

Variations: Substitute parsley leaves and stems for the basil, or use the parsley in combination with the basil, blending them together in the food processor. Or add a touch of stronger herbs, such as rosemary or sage to taste, to a parsley pesto. You can also replace the herbs above with cilantro, sorrel, arugula, or mint, adding a touch of fresh chives, if you like. Try local soft cheeses, such as fresh goat or ricotta, solo or in combination with a hard grating cheese. Or omit the cheese and try fresh lemon juice or hot chilies.

Serving suggestions: Spread on sandwiches or wraps; thin with a little cooking water and toss on pasta to coat; toss with roasted vegetables; stir into mayo, butter, or sauces (without the cheese); add to stuffings; or omit nuts and add to soup.

Herb Butter or Oil

Mix softened, unsweetened butter with chopped herbs to taste, adding a touch of salt, if you like. Roll in wax paper, twist the ends, mark, and freeze. For herb-scented oil, blend herbs with a flavorless oil or light olive oil, strain through a fine strainer, then add salt to taste.

Serving suggestions: Serve butter in thin slices, or melt it and drizzle on fish, chicken, meat, or vegetables.

Herb Persillade

Blend or chop together 2 cups parsley, cilantro, chervil, or dill with ⅓ cup olive oil and 2 garlic cloves.

Variation: Add a touch of grated lemon zest.

Serving suggestion: Sprinkle over or toss with any savory dish.

Italian Parsley Caper Sauce

Make parsley pesto, page 129, without the cheese or nuts. Blend in capers and lemon juice to taste.

Variation: Add a touch of Dijon mustard or anchovy paste.

Serving suggestions: This sauce is fabulous when served with fish, chicken, grilled eggplant, or mushrooms.

Fried Sage or Parsley Leaves

Batter and fry! Eat immediately.

Serving suggestions: Alone or as a garnish.

Dilled Horseradish

To yogurt, mayonnaise, crème fraiche, sour cream, or a combination of two, add freshly grated horseradish and dill to taste. Season with salt.

Serving suggestion: Great with fish, especially smoked fish.

Herb Croutons

Use fresh or stale bread cubes or torn pieces of bread. Toss them with just a touch of olive oil and herbs, such as rosemary. Season with salt and pepper to taste, if needed. Bake the cubes in a single layer on a baking sheet in a 400°F oven, shaking the pan occasionally until they are toasted.

Variation: Cook a small amount of cubes in a large sauté pan until brown, adding minced garlic, if you like, during the last minute or so of cooking so it doesn't burn.

Serving suggestion: Add to soups and salads.

Chimichurri Sauce

This sauce works best in a blender. Combine 1 cup packed parsley leaves, 1 minced garlic clove, and 1 very thinly sliced sweet onion. With the motor running, pour ¼ cup olive oil and up to ¼ cup water through the top hole. Add 1 tablespoon lime juice, 1 teaspoon white vinegar, and a generous pinch of sugar. Blend until smooth. Season with salt and freshly ground black pepper to taste.

Serving suggestions: Drizzle over fish, any kind of meat, or vegetables.

Starting with Turkey

Change can come all at once or one ingredient at a time. Try a real turkey this holiday, or anytime at all. Farm fresh turkeys are a different bird entirely from the standard factory-farmed frozen turkeys, which are raised as quickly as possible in tight living quarters. They're raised for their white meat and are often injected with a solution to make them juicier and more flavorful. Conventionally raised large birds can be moist and tender, but they can also be mushy or off-flavor. Breeds are chosen for commercial reasons only. The producers don't have the time or food necessary to develop great bird flavor.

Alternatively, farm-fresh turkeys bring with them a real story of your regional farm and can have a distinctive flavor as well. They're more expensive, but they are well worth it. You'll find two tiers on the expense ladder. On the less-expensive tier are regional turkeys that are fresh, not frozen. These may or may not be organic, and you should check with your farm about whether they use additives, antibiotics, or growth hormones. I've bought and enjoyed plenty of these.

Up the dollar ladder substantially are heritage turkeys, with breeds like Bourbon Reds that descended from the first turkeys in America. Heritage breeds (and sometimes conventional breeds) are allowed to roam freely and forage for some or all of their food. They have a deeper flavor and a firmer texture. And no additives, growth hormones, or antibiotics are added.

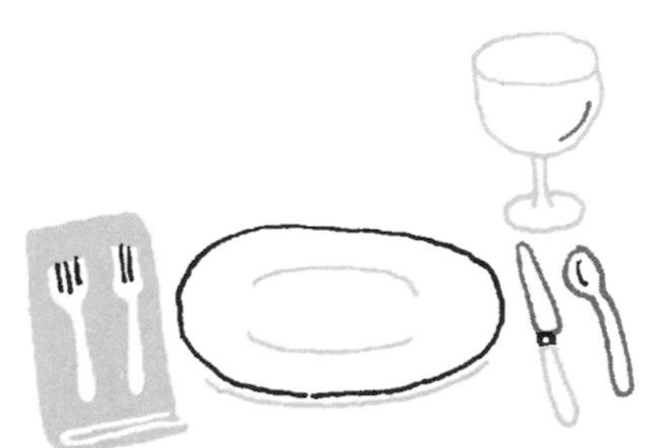

Note that organic birds, heritage breeds or not, are even more expensive, but some say they are well worth the outlay. Organic growers abide by a specific set of USDA rules. The turkeys have to be free of pesticides, growth hormones, antibiotics, and certain unnatural substances and processing techniques. They also have to be fed only organic feed. Having said that, if I have to choose, I generally choose local over organic.

If you're cooking a farm-fresh turkey, make sure you baste it, because it hasn't been injected with who-knows-what to make it juicy. Slather the turkey with butter, salt, and pepper, then set it upright in a 450°F oven on a rack for 15 minutes. Then lower the oven temperature to 350°F, basting the bird every 20 minutes with drippings, oil, or butter until a meat thermometer inserted into the thigh reads 180°F. To keep the breast from drying out, dip a cheesecloth in drippings or oil and rest it on top of the bird, adding oil if necessary. Once the turkey is browned, keep a little water in the bottom of the pan. Don't overcook! The timing is less reliable, but I also like to smoke my turkey over charcoal or wood, brined or as-is, on my Weber grill with the lid on and a small disposable pan of water underneath the bird.

Sadly, like so many, both of my local turkey farms went out of the turkey-raising business, but they still buy fresh birds from regional farms. Buying from these farms keeps them alive. I like to buy a big bird, because you can't beat the leftovers. In fact, we do a big turkey dinner several times a year, in part because I love to play with the leftovers and the flavorful turkey stock made from simmering the carcass. That stock cures any winter cold.

Dining Out

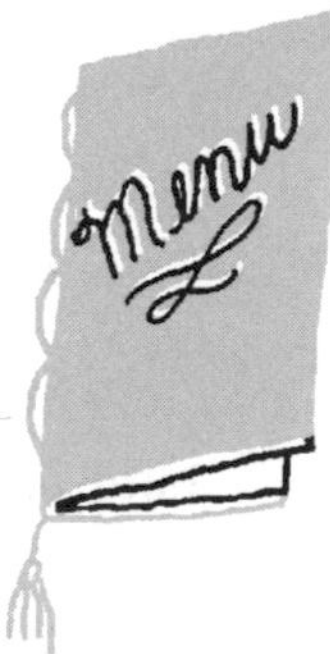

"Using local farm foods is selfish. We put better food on the plate because of it."

DAVID JAMES ROBINSON
Chef-Owner, Bezalel Gables Fine Catering, Chatham, New York

Going out to eat is one of the simplest ways to savor local foods and support the farmers that grew it. Restaurant chefs spearheaded the local food revolution, introducing seasonal goodies into their menus because they taste great. Around the country, they bought and served organic mesclun lettuce mix decades before it became mainstream. People enjoyed it out and drove the demand up. In the process, farmer-to-chef connections were forged. These matches resulted in long-term partnerships and, as importantly, magic on your plate when you dine out.

Still, it's often tough to find local or even regional food at restaurants. Chefs may know that local food is fresher, tastier, and comes from a more responsive purveyor, but buying locally can also add extra work and more expense. It's easier (and sometimes mandated) for chefs to order from just a few, or even one, supplier by phone or online than to develop multiple relationships with regional farmers or work with distributors who stock local foods. And seasonal buying can be tough, too. If the strawberry crop is wiped out by rain, do chefs order California berries or switch the dessert to whatever local fruit is available?

Despite these hurdles, a cadre of chefs nationwide is committed to presenting and preparing local food menus. Their efforts enable us to have a blast while doing the right thing, a rare combo. So open the door and walk into a restaurant that serves local food. Healing the food system may be complex, but dining out isn't.

TIPS FOR DINING OUT

Find 'em. Track down restaurants and take-out joints that serve local foods. This hunt can take some effort. But

A CUMULATIVE IMPACT

The number of meals eaten away from home has more than doubled in less than 30 years to more than one in three meals. These days, about 40 percent of the U.S. household food budget is spent on food eaten outside the home, with the average person eating out at least once a day. If even a small portion of the local $500 billion spent annually in restaurants was spent on local food, it would radically impact our food system — from increasing farm sales and lowering transport costs to bringing better, fresher food to the table.

once you find a few that serve local food, your work is done.

Try the direct route. You won't always get a satisfactory result over the phone, but before you decide whether to eat there, it's worth calling a restaurant and asking, "Do you serve local farm foods?" If possible, get them to be specific. What are they featuring on their menu now?

Ask a fellow locavore. Word of mouth can be magic.

Check the Chefs Collaborative Web site. You may be pleasantly surprised. (See Resources.)

Study the menu. On-site or Web-based menus can tip you off as to whether a business is likely to serve local food. Do they make it easy for you, bragging about it by mentioning farm names right on the menu? Interest in seasonal foods is another clue. Do they change their menus seasonally or at least feature specific dishes with seasonal produce at peak harvest, such as apple desserts in the fall and asparagus side dishes in the spring? Read carefully. Do entrees mention varieties of produce, such a Macoun apples, rather than generically listing foods? These items show that the kitchen has an interest in the singular taste of specific foods and may be interested in regional foods. Do they feature membership in any organization that supports sustainable agriculture?

Ask your farmer. Many sell to restaurants. While shopping at farmers' markets, farm stands, or CSAs, ask, "Is there anywhere I can get these delicious ingredients when I'm dining out?"

Get a helping hand. Tap into organizations that steer consumers to farm-friendly restaurants. Some are national, such as the Chefs Collaborative. Statewide, look for organizations such as Vermont Fresh Network (see Resources), or try the marketing division of your Department of Agriculture. Locally, check with your Chamber of Commerce or groups like Berkshire Grown near me (see Resources). This plan of action works well when you're visiting from out of town, too.

Don't dismiss budget eateries. I love an honest meal — truly fresh foods cooked simply and well. What I enjoy most is the inherent magic when great ingredients are prepared without a fuss. So when eating out, I'm an equal opportunity pleasure seeker. I'm not surprised to find delicious food in roadside diners, ethnic family spots, or elegant white-tablecloth restaurants. While local food is often associated with fine dining — because higher end restaurants tend to have more skilled labor and a larger budget — don't dismiss lower-budget places that may care deeply about food quality and have special arrangements with a local farmer. I've had a silky butternut squash soup at my local breakfast-all-day restaurant, Martin's, where the owner buys his squash — as well as other inexpensive items, like zucchini and corn — when it's in season, from nearby Taft Farms. He doesn't make a big deal of it, but it's part of what he does.

Chain restaurants and fast food joints are much tougher. Most don't serve local foods, although there are some exceptions, like an independently owned regional burger chain with a local grass-fed burger option. And corporations such as Chipotle plan to require their 700-plus restaurants to buy a percentage of their produce from local farms. More are likely to pop up.

Local food can transform the simplest meal out into something memorable — a fresh slab of tomato on a grass-fed burger, a salad of lively greens with local cheese and fall apples, or corn chowder that's shockingly fresh.

WHEN YOU GET THERE, ASK

Make a habit of always asking your server, "What's local?" on the menu whenever you eat out. You may come up empty or be pleasantly surprised. But asking sends a message to the food buyer (most often the chef, if it's an independently owned restaurant): customers want local food! If your initial answer is no, ask your server to check with the kitchen, because a chef using local foods may not clue in his

THE CHEFS COLLABORATIVE

Chefs brought the local food movement to the front burner for customers who savored local food at their restaurants. And Chefs Collaborative — a national nonprofit supporting sustainable agriculture whose membership is primarily culinary professionals — has led the way. The Collaborative teaches chefs how to do it right, and they work with kindred organizations on other sustainable and local-food-based projects. Visit their Web site (see Resources) for communiqués, clearly written pieces unraveling food issues, and for a list of member restaurants focused on local and sustainable foods. One may be located near you!

or her wait staff. If this happens and you discover a great dish, your servers will know next time they're asked; they may even recommend it.

ORDER LOCAL FOODS

If you don't order them, they won't stay on the menu. Even a small percentage of people ordering local foods — say, cheese soufflé in the winter or the heirloom tomato salad in the summer — may help support a small neighboring farm.

Scan the menu for farm foods you know are locally available already from your locavore's shopping or produce charts (follow the Web link for Sustainable Table in Resources). That way, when you spot corn in season, you can ask, "Is it local?" Or if you know

Ice Cream Goes Local

I fell in love with Jeni's Ice Cream at her stand in Columbus, Ohio's North Market which is brimming with lively local food businesses and a weekly farmers' market.

A passion for local foods often starts with flavor, and owner Jeni Britton's unctuous ice cream is top-notch. Her signature ice cream, Salty Caramel, with its surprising play of salty-sweet, was my first try.

"Anything that grows, you can put in ice cream," says Jeni, from familiar ingredients like strawberries to off-beat cucumbers, sweet potatoes, and the roasted Kabocha winter squash used in her flavor, Winter Squash with Pecan Pralines. Some of her ice creams are sweetened with local honey and maple syrup; one is seasoned with local spicebush berries, similar to allspice.

Jeni serves a trio of little scoops, a boon to the ice cream lover. Her favorite farm-fresh combination is: Strawberry Rose Petal, Honey Vanilla Bean, and Goat Cheese. All of her distinctive flavors are carried by the milk she uses.

"I'm obsessed with quality milk," Jeni says. "Although it's hard to find local milk sources here, and we've switched several times, I see a huge difference in milk produced from small regional dairies. It is creamier in color and flavor, far better than in commodity milk. We're working toward our goal of producing our ice cream right on the dairy farm. Although some food policies make this hard, I know we'll get there."

Menu Savvy

"I always look at a restaurant menu before I make a reservation, to quickly get a sense if they use local produce, and it's worth the effort. If you're in the Northeast and see mangos and asparagus in July or August, then you aren't getting what the region has to offer."

DAN BARBER

Blue Hill and Blue Hill at Stone Barns, Manhattan and Pocantico Hills, New York

FOOD SERVICE GETS SMART

Although still not the norm, some food service corporations, notably Bon Appetít Management Company, emphasize local food-buying practices. So when you're dining at an institution, in a corporate dining room, and especially at a museum or college dining hall, look for and ask about local food. And why not try to get your executive dining room or workplace cafeteria to buy local foods?

about a great regional cheese, you can ask for it. Drinks — particularly wine, beer, hard liquor, and even apple cider — are often the easiest local items to find on the menu.

Restaurants using regional meat, poultry, or fish often boast about it on their menu, especially if it is sustainably raised or caught. (Note that good food isn't cheap to produce. Restaurant margins are slim, so consider paying a little more to order the good stuff.)

And don't forget to order local ingredients already integrated into dishes, such as value-added products like maple syrup or honey used in a dessert, wine in a sauce, or fruit in a salad. There may be local eggs or nuts in a cake. The milk for your coffee might come from the neighboring dairy and, if you are lucky, the ice cream as well. Beverages like juice and even water may be local, too, so ask again if you don't see an attribution on the menu.

GIVE FEEDBACK

Your server asks, "Did you enjoy your meal?" If you did, answer that you especially enjoyed the local ____ and fill in the blank. Send compliments to the chef for making the effort to serve the best local fare. Or if nothing was local, express your disappointment in any way that feels natural to you, including, "The meal was lovely, but tomatoes are in season, and I would have enjoyed ripe local tomatoes in my salad."

SPREAD THE WORD

Once you've struck gold, spread the word to family and friends to patronize this restaurant. And, as you've already done the homework, tell them what you found that was tasty on the menu.

MAKE A MATCH IF YOU COME UP EMPTY

You may not find a restaurant near you that serves local foods. But keep asking, as this may change and it also helps to create demand. Get to know a restaurant chef and farm vendor you patronize, then offer to help make a farm match that works for both. Deliver brochures from a local food or farm advocacy group or work with them to encourage farm-to-fork connections in your community. (See page 198.)

Beyond Restaurants

While eating foods available close to home has been the norm since cavemen chomped on their first mammoth, current advocates for local food consumption are pegged as an elitist crowd for a variety of reasons — some real, some imagined. (See Fight Hunger with Local Food Democracy on page 202.) It's a sore point with some of us farm-to-table advocates, and it seems particularly irksome that everyday foods are often not made with local products. Take the hot dog, often the butt (yes, that too) of jokes about what's in them. Which is one of the reasons I so adore local items like ice cream and hot dogs.

USE A CATERER WHO FEATURES LOCAL FOODS ON THE MENU

Bezalel Gables Fine Catering is located in Chatham, New York, in a stunning Queen Anne Victorian, surrounded by hundreds of acres of farmland. Chef-Owner David James Robinson specializes in high-end pastry as well as artisan-made foods from local farms. Everything is made from scratch, including house-cured and smoked salmon, fresh and smoked mozzarella, and his pride and joy, vanilla ice cream, churned from local milk and eggs.

"People can go to The Gap anywhere and get the same music and same clothes. But if they come to Hudson Valley, they want to eat food from the ground they stand on, something with a sense of place," says David.

When planning a catered event, why not ask for local food on your menu? For the most part, you'll find a locavore-friendly caterer the same way you find a restaurant that serves local food (see Find 'em on page 134). Of course, it's easiest to start by hiring a caterer who already uses local foods.

Live in wine country or visiting? Eat out at a winery overlooking a vineyard that serves its own wine paired with local foods, like artisanal cheeses.

Hot Dogs

"Our hot dogs are my haiku for the food system:
everything you need to know about a healthy food system contained on the bun."
— Larry Bain, Co-Owner of Let There Be Frank, a natural hot dog business

Let There Be Frank partners Larry Bain (farm-to-table activist and self-titled "head weenie") and Sue Moore (meat forager for Chez Panisse) produce a hot dog using free-range, grass-fed beef from the reasonably local Hearst Farm in San Simeon, California.

The idea came naturally. Chez Panisse was butchering two head of cattle every other week for the restaurant, and Sue wanted to use the trimmings. Voilà: dogs. While you may have unpleasant images of the kind of animal extras used in hot dogs, these dogs use cuts normally found in pot roast, steak sandwiches, or brisket.

After trying dozens of recipes, they came up with a winning wiener — a meaty, rich-tasting, all-natural dog. It's a meat-colored dog (not fluorescent pink, as some dogs are), cured with celery seed extract rather than nitrates and nitrites, lower in salt and fat, spiced with garlic and paprika, and packaged in a lamb casing.

The dogs are a culturally accessible local food made from healthy, sustainably raised, grass-fed meat. What's just as exciting is that they're a universally affordable local food for everyone. Condiments include locally made organic sauerkraut and an Acme bakery organic bun. Order the works, and with sales tax, it's about five bucks.

The first audience for Let There Be Frank hot dogs was all-American — the ballpark in San Francisco. There Sue quickly learned to stress the dogs' good flavor rather than their health benefits, filling people in only when they asked. After all, who goes to a game for the health food? Mostly served by Sue, the dogs are available at San Francisco baseball home games and at Crissey field. The goal is to have a few carts located around San Francisco and Los Angeles, have them available at mom-and-pop stores, and eventually get into bigger venues, too.

Let There Be Frank aims to preserve the few ranches who are engaged in pasture-based livestock management operations and to encourage those who are now using feedlots to transition to grass.

But if you can't find one, steer your caterer toward local food sources you already know about. Who knows? You may end up introducing them to the whole idea of eating locally.

When making menu arrangements long before your party, be flexible about the produce so your caterer can nail it down closer to the event. This way, they use what's coming in best that season: asparagus may usually arrive in June, for example, but what if it's a cold spring and the asparagus season will be starting late? When I catered, I usually put "seasonal local vegetables" on the menu. Then I picked up the best of the harvest, discussing it with my clients, if necessary, a week or so before the event so we could agree on the selection.

And of course, this isn't just about produce, so be sure to ask about everything from meat and fish, depending on where you live, to dairy products such as cheeses, milk, and eggs. My neighbor, Jeremy Stanton of Fire Roasted Catering in Sheffield, Massachusetts, whole smokes heritage pork right on the premises. And it isn't difficult to add regional milk or cheese to any menu.

After you agree on a menu, be very clear about what you expect to be local. Note that some caterers may charge a small premium for adding a more expensive local item to your menu. If that squeezes your budget too much, maybe you can eliminate something else, like a choice of desserts. Better to have less choice and higher quality.

A Sampling of Winter Menus

SAVOY
New York City, New York

Vermont suckling pig roulade, red and white cabbage, smoked spaetzle and Bosc pears

L'ETOILE
Madison, Wisconsin

Pan-roasted Grass is Greener chicken with Fantôme Farm chèvre, Black Earth Valley mushroom and Delicata squash risotto, braised Harmony Valley escarole

GIBBET GRILL HILL
Groton, Massachusetts

Meatloaf, country glazed carrots, garlic mashed potatoes, rich mushroom-bacon gravy

Fine Dining, the Locavore Way

"Our guests overlook a field of growing tomatoes, so it's not hard to examine seasonal food issues. Our canvas is right in people's faces."

DAN BARBER

Blue Hill at Stone Barns, Pocantico Hills, New York

Dan Barber takes the local food revolution to the next level in his luxury restaurant, Blue Hill at Stone Barns within Stone Barns Center for Food and Agriculture in Pocantico Hills, New York.

Guests drive past a sweeping farm and educational center dotted with grazing heritage sheep. A stroll by the kitchen garden, brimming with vegetables and flowers, takes them to an unadorned dining room, overlooking the herbal tea garden and farm. There, Dan, executive chef and co-owner, provides the ultimate farm-to-table experience by serving food in its context — on the farm.

Rather than a menu, diners order from an ingredient list of the season's bounty, which serves as the chef's palette. The ordering process teases out the diner's tastes and expectations. By way of explanation, the waitstaff may bring raw farm ingredients to the table. After ordering, guests are asked to sit back and give their trust to the kitchen staff, as they turn out 10 to 15 variations on these core ingredients. Entrees can be as cautious as a pork chop or as edgy as a snout. Dishes like Potato and Green Garlic Ravioli rely on the ingredients' distinctive flavor and freshness.

Dan has built his reputation on emphasizing sustainably raised farm foods. It's a calculated risk; some diners can't understand why they are served certain varieties of summer green beans or why any crop at its seasonal peak appears repeatedly in the same meal. And sustainable cooking can be especially challenging when it comes to meat. Like other eco-conscious chefs, Dan has bucked the tradition of ordering only prime cuts, instead using as much of the animal as he can. After 16 pork chops, that's it for one pig, so diners are presented with more braised dishes. There are also out-of-the-norm dishes, such as fried lamb's brains — a crisp nugget with a soft center — or roasted marrow — served right out of the lower shank of a cow. These, along with harvest dishes such as classic heirloom tomato salads and farm-raised chicken in a sauce of fresh peas and morel mushrooms, make the farm-to-fork connection deliciously.

OUT ON THE FARM

Stone Barns Center for Food and Agriculture sits on 80 acres, donated by David Rockefeller, just 45 minutes north of Manhattan. It houses the restaurant, farm, and educational center, which teaches and advocates for locally based food production and enjoyment. The latter two are free and open to the public.

Although the complex has an almost air-brushed, utopian look, Stone Barns Center operates as a nonprofit. Its sweeping landscape centers on

A PEEK AT THE AUGUST MENU OFFERINGS AT BLUE HILL AT STONE BARNS

From the Greenhouse

buttercrunch lettuce • Ruby Red chard • Red Russian kale • Mokum carrots • Pirat lettuce • arugula • golden purslane • Italian parsley • Malibar spinach • mizuna • tatsoi

From the Field

black currants • Sweet Chocolate peppers • squash blossoms • bay leaves • arcuri garlic • Royal Burgundy string beans • cauliflower • Cherokee Purple tomatoes • broccoli • lemongrass • round picante squash • Tuscan Black kale • Prosperosa eggplant • pineapple sage • 66 more freshly harvested foods . . .

the restored stone, wood, and steel buildings, which sit around a courtyard, once the site of the Rockefellers' dairy operation and now home to a farmers' market three times a week. The diversified organic farm sells 60 percent of its bounty to the restaurant and the remainder at the market.

The farm grows 200 varieties of in-ground and greenhouse produce. In September, heirloom tomatoes in a spectrum of warm colors hang heavy on the vine with baskets at each row's end filled to the brim. The grounds bustle with livestock and poultry — a multitude of egg-laying and meat-producing chickens, Finn-Dorset sheep, and Berkshire pigs with their leatherlike skins. Bourbon Red heritage turkeys, known for their complex flavor, nest in the trees at night.

"The luxuries at Blue Hill are white tomatoes and heritage pig, not foie gras and lobster," Dan says.

For more information about the center and other on-farm educational programs, see Resources.

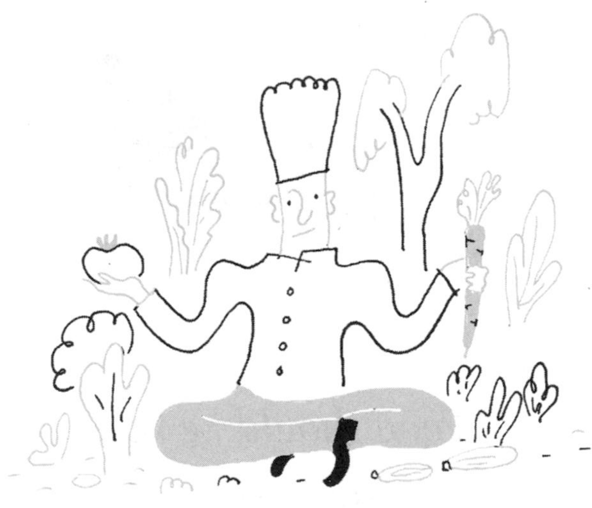

Play with Your Produce

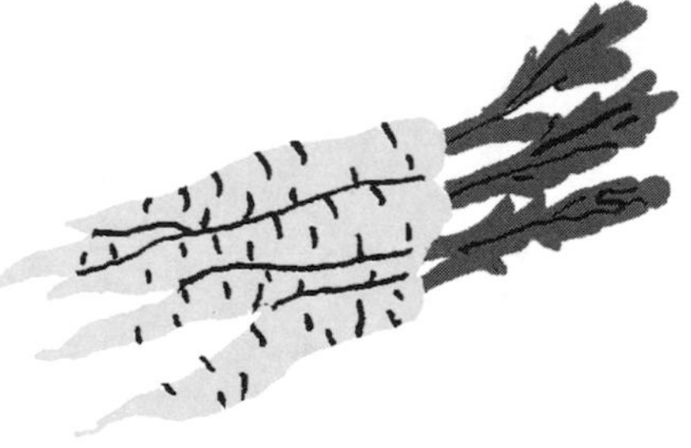

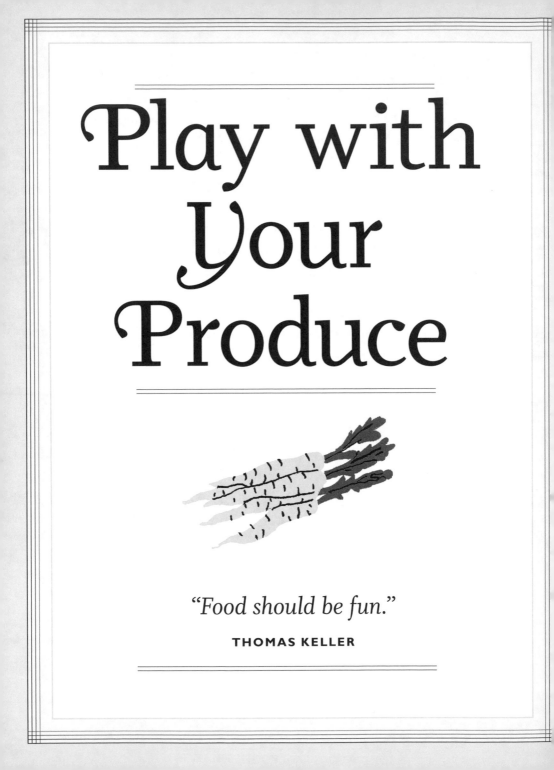

"Food should be fun."

THOMAS KELLER

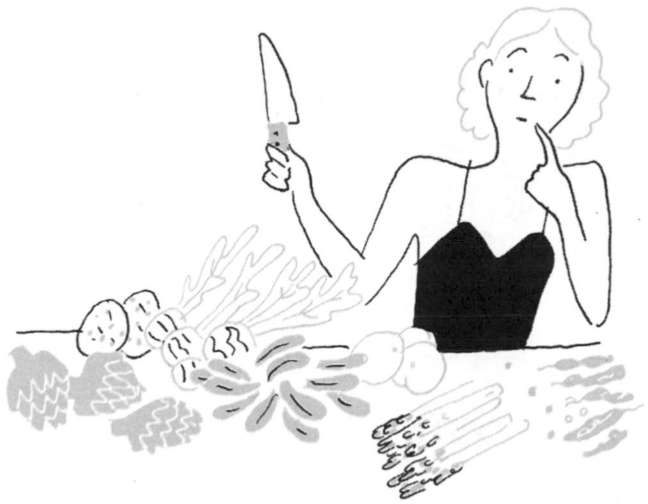

What should you do with the harvest? Here's a produce riff, ideas for the novice or experienced cook, a resource to refer to either before or after you shop. When you have the chance, be sure to try varieties that aren't widely available in the supermarket. You'll be astounded at the flavor differences. If you keep to my less-is-more theory of local food cooking, letting the food star and not fussing too much, you can't lose. While this section focuses on produce, general information about other ingredients starts on page 166. Directions on how to store produce begins on page 104.

Now you have no excuses; you have plenty of ideas for ways to play with your local produce. And of course, these are just the tip of the iceberg. Now go to it!

NEED A HELPING HAND?

Take a quick look at the improvisational tips and techniques on page 114 to refresh your memory. If you're still feeling a little lost, use the ideas here as a source of inspiration, adapting them to recipes from cookbooks or online. (Even pros do this!) If you want to go further, get an overview of general cooking techniques, such as frying, grilling, and more on my Web site (see Resources). And finally, never underestimate the power of salt to bring out the flavor in your veggies!

Remember that the simplest and often the most delicious way to savor local food is to eat it raw and whole, like a freshly picked apple.

Let the Ingredients Star

Local food doesn't require much of you. All you have to do is let your ingredients star by allowing their flavor to shine. So keep it simple. Crunch on crisp apples and peeled carrots; bite into a juicy peach. Steam broccoli lightly and toss it in a touch of fruity olive oil, a squeeze of lemon, and a pinch of salt rather than mixing it with a thousand different flavors. If you're not experienced with seasoning, try new flavors one by one, adding each to various dishes before combining it with other flavors. Add one, two, or at the most a trilogy of flavors at first — such as butter, shallots, and wine for a French feel or soy, ginger, and scallions for an Asian touch. Just as too many colors mix into brown, too many flavors result in a muddy flavor. Be sure you're adding flavors for the role they'll play, not simply to add them. (I see too many recipes loaded down with unnecessary seasonings.) Try combinations that contrast (mild cauliflower with hot curry), highlight classic compatibility (potatoes and rosemary), or are simply fun, but don't disguise the flavor of the food itself with too much.

The key to becoming a good improvisational cook is to use all your senses. The food gives you clues through its fragrance, look, and taste. Use those clues to guide you, and remember them (or write them down for) next time around.

APPLES

Do a taste test of different varieties, to see just how unique each one is. ■ Slice and serve with local cheese. ■ Bake classic crisps, tarte tatins, pies, tarts, or free-form galettes (which are especially easy to make). ■ For baked apples, core, fill with what pleases you, then bake in a little cider until soft. Ideal fillings are any combination of cinnamon, maple syrup, honey or jam, nuts and dried fruit, or butter. ■ For better-than-you-can-imagine warm applesauce, quarter apples without peeling or coring, simmer until very soft, then put through a food mill; add spice, if you like. Good in baked goods, too. ■ Roast with root vegetables to use in pureed soups. ■ Toss in salads with bitter greens, like escarole.

APRICOTS

Halve, pit, and slice; then simmer, sweetened to taste, with a dash of your favorite alcohol, such as amaretto or brandy. Serve as-is with local ice cream or yogurt. ■ Great in tarts or jam.

ARTICHOKE

The versatile artichoke can be steamed, fried, sautéed, or braised. It loves garlic, lemon, and olive oil. ■ Serve it whole, as-is, or stuffed. ■ Dip the warm leaves, then heart, in melted butter or marinate the whole thing overnight in a garlicky oil-and-vinegar dressing. ■ Serve the raw inner hearts thinly sliced in a salad, or stuff and bake them. ■ Enjoy the tasty stems, ends removed and well peeled, or chop and add them to a stuffing. ■ To braise raw artichoke wedges, cut off two-thirds of the leaves, cut the artichoke lengthwise into eighths, remove the fuzzy choke, sauté with seasonings such as onions and garlic, then

THE SIMPLEST WAY TO STEAM A WHOLE ARTICHOKE

Cut off the top inch of the leaves with a sharp or heavy serrated knife. (Remove the stem, peel it, and steam it with the rest of the artichoke, but for less time. It is delicious.) Steam in a couple of inches of water (adding lemon and garlic, if desired), with or without a steamer, for 25 to 40 minutes or until you can remove a leaf easily. Remove the bottom row or two of leaves. Insert a spoon into the center to gently remove the choke, or have diners remove their own. Serve warm with melted butter, or cool with a garlicky dressing.

Optional: If you want to trim an artichoke more professionally before cooking, bend and snap off the bottom row of leaves, until only the whitish tender portion remains. Trim around the base with a knife, rubbing with lemon as you go to prevent discoloring. With scissors, cut off the tips of the remaining leaves. If you like, you can remove the inner fuzzy choke before cooking, especially if you plan on stuffing it.

braise covered with a little water over medium heat until tender.

ARUGULA

see Salad Greens

ASPARAGUS

Snap off the end of one stalk. Loosely line the rest up and chop them off all at about the same place. Or if you have time, snap each individually, or cut off the bottom inch and peel the bottom third of the stalk. ■ Use the plunge-and-dress technique on page 116. Serve with butter and Parmesan cheese or in a vinaigrette — a dressing with 3 parts oil to 1 part vinegar or lemon. ■ It's just as good blanched briefly, oiled slightly, and then grilled or roasted. ■ Try battered and deep fried, too!

AVOCADO

Halve and remove the pit, then spoon out the flesh. Mash into guacamole, or dice into salads. Either way, add acid — such as citrus juice or vinegar — to prevent browning. ■ If not slightly soft to the touch, ripen in a brown bag for a few days. ■ In this country, Haas avocados, with their pebbly skins, are mostly grown in California. The smooth-skinned Fuerte is less common.

BEANS AND LEGUMES, DRIED OR FRESH

The numerous varieties of fresh and dried beans all have different flavors, so experiment.

Fresh green, yellow, or purple beans respond well to the plunge-and-dress technique (see page 116). Or skip the dressing and wok with garlic and oil, Asian seasoning, or nuts. ■ Try long, slow, Italian-style braising with seasonings and/or meat. ■ Petite haricot verts have a delicate flavor, so they're best when lightly steamed. ■ Try fabulous favas; they're an effort to shell, though, so start with dinner for one or two.

Dried beans (and legumes) make terrific salads, soups, stews, and side dishes. They can be cooked without soaking, but take longer. Either way, fill a pot of water 2 inches above the beans, cover and simmer until cooked, checking occasionally to see if extra water is needed. Season during or after cooking, but add salt last and be generous. ■ Beans love a touch of acid from tomatoes or vinegar, garlic, as well as Mediterranean or south-of-the-border flavors.

BEETS

Roasted beets are a great staple. ■ Trim greens, leaving a bit of the stem. (To cook greens, see page 157.) Wrap beets in foil, and roast in a 400°F oven until soft all the way through (poke with a knife). When cool, slip off skins and stems.

Slice, julienne, or grate cooked beets to serve as a side or salad. They love dressing or just a toss of balsamic or other vinegar. ■ Top salads with grated raw beets. ■ Serve cooked beets alone or with a combination of other dressed vegetables (two or four of contrasting colors), each separated on the plate for a pretty composed salad. ■ Or serve with a green salad with local goat cheese, toasted nuts, or fruit. ■ Blend roasted beets with buttermilk, a drop of balsamic, salt, and pepper for an easy cold summer borscht. Top with sour cream and chives. ■ Make a traditional, colorful, beet ravioli.

BERRIES

Make a float, as owner-chef Peter Hoffman does at Savoy in New York City, with local ice cream, slightly crushed berries, cassis, and bubbly water. ■ Make a berry crisp, adding a little fresh ground pepper or nuts to the topping. ■ Sprinkle berries into fruit salads at the last minute. ■ Assemble parfaits with local yogurt, using raw or very slightly sautéed berries sweetened with sugar, local maple syrup or honey, and touch of kirsch or a local liqueur, layered with ice cream or whipped cream. ■ Experiment with unfamiliar berries, like gooseberries, blackberries, or loganberries. ■ Add blueberries to classic muffins and pies. ■ Go savory: Sprinkle berries in green salads or throw them into a meat sauté at the last minute. ■ Serve a raspberry-nut dressing with greens by lightly cooking local nuts in flavorless oil to make a nut oil, then tossing with raspberries and a touch of vinegar.

BROCCOLI

Cut into bite-sized florets. You can also use the stem, if you wish: discard the tough end, peel the rest with a sharp knife, and then thinly slice on the diagonal. Cook the sliced stem pieces with florets or reserve them for a stir-fry. ■ Plunge and shock (see page 115), or plunge but don't shock and dress with olive oil and lemon, or a light toss of soy, freshly grated ginger, a drop or two of sesame oil, and scallions. ■ Use the plunge, shock, and dress method for all kinds of salads. ■ Use the plunge-and-dress pasta technique (see page 116), throwing in the peeled, sliced stems a minute or two before the florets. Dress as you like, or toss with garlic oil, hot chili pepper flakes, and Parmesan. ■ Broccoli is also popular simmered until soft in creamed soups and cooked into quiches.

BROCCOLI RABE

see Greens, Cooking

BRUSSELS SPROUTS

My sister calls them parakeet heads, but I continue to insist that they're fabulous when cooked right. Cut off the ends, but not so much that they fall apart. (You're supposed to make an X with a knife on the bottoms so they cook evenly, but I seldom do.) Steam just until tender all the way through but still bright. Season with butter that's been cooked until slightly brown and nutty in flavor. ■ Halve them, toss them in oil and seasonings (if you like), arrange them in a single layer on a baking sheet, and roast them at 400°F. Add peeled and halved shallots or sautéed onions and pancetta. They're done when you taste one and like it.

CABBAGE

This is truly an underrated vegetable! Enjoy it in vegetable soups, such as bistro-style cabbage and potato soup: just shred and simmer in broth and sprinkle with blue cheese. ■ Make a fresh coleslaw: grate or thinly slice red or green cabbage, then toss with your favorite dressing (I like an Asian-flavored one); try adding colorful grated carrots or even butternut squash. ■ Use the plunge-and-dress pasta technique (see page 116), adding sliced cabbage during the last 3 minutes of cooking, then tossing with butter, salt, pepper, and a touch of caraway seeds. ■ Make sweet-and-sour style cabbage by braising it in a covered pot with a little vinegar, local sweetener (such as honey or maple syrup), salt, and pepper; serve with roasted local poultry. ■ Make homemade sauerkraut with caraway, which tastes miles above the packaged stuff. ■ Try all types of cabbages: Napa, Savoy, and the more common green and red cabbages. And don't forget the Asian varieties, such as Chinese bok choy, both white and green. All are great when stir-fried briefly with two or more Asian seasonings, such as ginger, scallions, soy, and sesame oil.

CARROTS

Slice (on the bias is pretty), cube, or julienne (long strips), then use the plunge-and-dress method (see page 116) with melted butter and a touch of fresh oregano or dill. ■ Grate raw for a salad, or to pickle with ginger, adapting a sauerkraut recipe. ■ Cube and add to any kind of grain dish, from brown rice to bulgur, throwing carrots in during the last 5 to 10 minutes of cooking. ■ Toast your favorite Indian spices, like curry or cumin, then add them to sliced carrots simmering in broth; puree into soup.

CARDOON

Unusual in this country, the cardoon is related to the artichoke, and it tastes a bit like an artichoke with a hint of celery. The edible part is the large stalk, not the flower head. Smaller stalks are the most tender, sometimes tender enough to eat raw as the Italians do, dipped in *bagna cauda* (a mix of olive oil and anchovy). ■ Cut stalks and plunge them into water with a touch of acid, such as lemon or vinegar, to prevent browning. Peel the pieces, removing any strings. Often stalks are boiled briefly before being added to dishes, as you would an artichoke heart. ■ Try it in a stewed or braised dish.

CAULIFLOWER

Steam, sauté, deep fry, or toss and roast. ■ This white relative of broccoli has a gentler flavor and so enjoys assertive Indian spices or mellower garlic butter and toasted breadcrumbs. ■ A stunning relative, Romanesco, has a compact head like a cauliflower, a lime green color, and florets that look like spiraling cones. Its flavor is more delicate than a cauliflower. Cook as you would cauliflower.

CELERY

Keep chilled stalks in water in the fridge. ■ Combine with green onion for a classic southern combination. ■ Braise in stock for a classic accompaniment to roasts. ■ Outer stalks are best for cooking; inner stalks add crunchy character to salads of all kinds. ■ The magic combination of cooked celery, carrots, and onion is a superb base in soups and stews.

CELERY ROOT (CELERIAC)

This delicious root vegetable is not to be missed! Thoroughly peel off every bit of the funky, knobby skin before preparing it. ■ Grate raw and toss in a remoulade mayonnaise for a bistro-style side salad or appetizer. ■ Cube and use the toss-and-roast technique (see page 117) with other root vegetables as-is or with meat or poultry. ■ For soup, simmer in broth with potatoes, parsnips (and a touch of garlic, if you like) then blend, adding cream, if desired. ■ Simmer as you would for mashed or smashed potatoes. (See Smashed Potatoes and Celery Root with Chives on page 121.)

CHARD

see Greens, Cooking

CHERRIES

Pit and sauté with any sweetener and a touch of your favorite alcohol; serve over local ice cream or with yogurt, igniting it if you like. ■ Make clafouti (custard dessert), ice cream, or shockingly good real cherry pie. ■ If you find sour cherries, try them! Store

Celeriac

"I have given celeriac — that big, knobby, and dare I say, ugly, vegetable as a gift — with a pretty bow tied around the neck or stem, along with a recipe card giving instructions for celery root soup or smashed celeriac (similar to mashed potatoes). People always get a kick out of the surprise element, as well as the gussied up packaging, and the humor seems to help open up their minds about the possibility of actually preparing and eating the thing!"

LUISA GARRETT

Pacific Coast Farmers' Market Association Market Manager, San Jose, California in liquor; make jam, jelly, chutney, or Hungarian sour cherry soup. ■ Freeze for cooking in the winter.

CHICORIES

I adore the crunch and bitter flavor of all kinds of chicory-related plants, including frisee, escarole, and curly endive. Serve by itself as a salad, with apple or pear, or with gentler greens; add a dressing that matches its vigorous flavor. ■ For a warm salad, heat sturdy chicories briefly and serve with a dressing. ■ Cook escarole as you would cooking greens (see page 157). ■ Use the pasta plunge-and-dress technique (see page 116) with garlic oil, fresh lemon juice, and lots of fresh pepper. ■ Cut bright radicchio into wedges, then brush with olive oil and grill. (See also Salad Greens on page 163 and Greens, Cooking on page 157.)

COLLARDS

see Greens, Cooking

CORN

You can't beat husked corn, with sweet butter, salt, and pepper, steamed or boiled for 3 minutes. ■ To grill, remove the silk but not the husks, and then soak before grilling. Or for a deeper smoke, grill husked ears directly. ■ To remove kernels, husk, remove the silk, then slice down the length of the cob with a sharp knife. ■ Use kernels in soups or stews, such as corn chowder with the Southwest flavor of cilantro and garden chilies, or with tomatoes and any garden herb. ■ Steam or microwave kernels for a minute, then add into any kind of vegetable, grain, or cooked dried bean dish. ■ Make tomato-corn salsa or soup. ■ Prepare corn pudding, corn bread (with kernels), or classic succotash with fresh lima beans.

CRANBERRIES

For a relish or sauce, sweeten to taste then cook until soft or chop in the food processor raw. ■ Cranberries make great additions to baked goods and savory sauces because of their tang.

CUCUMBERS

These are especially tasty the day they are harvested. ■ Try dense, flavorful varieties like kirbys and Armenian cukes. ■ Peel and slice, or cut into spears. If they are very seedy, cut in half lengthwise and scoop out seeds with a spoon before slicing. ■ Use cuke slices as a base for a last minute canapé. ■ Dice and toss with a sprinkling of salt, let drain for 20 minutes to 1 hour in the fridge, then toss again with yogurt and vinegar to coat, adding touch of chopped sweet onion or scallion and a dash of dill. Great with pita triangles or to accompany lamb.

EGGPLANT

Available in various sizes and shapes — I especially enjoy skinny Japanese eggplant — all kinds of eggplant take similar cooking techniques. ■ Pierce a few times with a fork, roast eggplant whole, uncovered, until quite soft, 20 minutes to 1 hour at 400°F (grill whole for a smoky taste). Or split and steam for a silky texture. When done, split and scoop out flesh, discard skin and seeds. Make an eggplant "caviar" by chopping or mashing the flesh with olive oil, garlic, and other ingredients, such as diced tomato, lemon juice, and fresh herbs. ■ Blend steamed flesh into baba ghanoush or grilled flesh into smoky eggplant soup. ■ Dice and sauté in a summer stew, caponata, or an Asian-flavored dish.

Try slicing, then brushing with oil and grilling until soft (see page 117). Use grilled slices for a tasty veggie antipasto, a no-fry eggplant Parmesan, or in a sandwich with garlic-basil oil and tomatoes or sesame mayonnaise and bitter greens. ■ Roll and stuff grilled eggplant slices, or layer with ingredients like local cheese, tomatoes, and basil. ■ Fry slices and add to any number of dishes.

Although it's still open to debate, many people feel that eggplant is less bitter when it's peeled and salted before cooking. All agree that salting keeps eggplant from absorbing too much oil. If you salt, blot dry before cooking.

FENNEL

Fennel's crisp bulb has a light licorice flavor, which mellows considerably when cooked. ■ Remove stem ends, reserving the leaves to chop and use as an herb. ■ Use young bulbs whole or remove outer layers if they seem tough. ■ Serve, either raw or cooked, chopped, sliced, or julienned in salads. ■ Terrific in risotto, soup, or stew with seafood, or simply tossed with freshly cooked shrimp with lemon and a fruity olive oil. ■ Simmer wedges until tender, toss with olive oil, skewer and grill until lightly browned. ■ Very thinly slice raw fennel bulbs for a simple salad with olive oil and thinly shaved Parmesan on top. ■ Excellent pickled (see page 126) or stewed.

FIGS

There are several kinds of figs to try; whichever you buy, they are best when eaten within a few days of purchase. ■ Cut into a tangy green salad or simple fruit salad. ■ Halve and fill with local goat cheese or any kind of blue cheese. Bake in tarts or use in savory sauces.

GINGER

Classic in Asian foods, the ginger rhizome adds a distinctive spicy flavor.

Although it is commonly peeled, I learned from Barbara Tropp's Chinese cookbook to use it as-is. I generally grate it to flavor oils, stir-fries, or vegetable dishes.

GRAPEFRUIT

see Oranges

GRAPES

Try all the different grape varieties, and don't shy away from those with seeds, as they tend to have better flavor. ■ Sauté with farm-raised poultry, or simply halve and throw into fruit or savory salads. ■ And of course, serve with cheese!

GREENS, COOKING

see also Salad Greens

Robust greens include collard, kale, dandelion, mustard, turnip, and broccoli rabe in the mustard family. Milder greens include spinach and Swiss chard. ■ To cook them up quickly, see page 124. ■ Try hearty, long-cooked, old-fashioned southern-style greens simmered with water and smoked pork or bacon. ■ All flavorful greens, such as collards and kale, like a touch of vinegar and plenty of salt; spinach enjoys a hint of nutmeg. ■ Greens are great baked into savory custards such as quiches and added at the last minute to soups, stews, and stir-fries.

HERBS

Adding just one kind of freshly chopped herb to a plain dish can produce miraculously delicious food. ■ Start by using herbs one at a time, so you'll understand what they do, then try combining them. Try these classic combinations: rosemary with potatoes or chicken, fennel fronds and fish, dill and cucumber. Move from there to pairs such as chives (oniony) with parsley (a bright green flavor), while never underestimating their power on their own. ■ Use fragile herb leaves, such as parsley, chervil, cilantro, tarragon, and dill in salads. If you want to keep their bright flavor and color, add to cooked dishes just before serving. ■ Use piney rosemary, perfumey sage, and aromatic thyme sparingly, as they are strong. ■ Try less commonly found herbs such as epazote, garlic chives, lemon balm, verbena, and sorrel. ■ Use herbs, especially those in the mint family, for fabulous infusions and teas (see pages 129–131 for preparation ideas, 109 and 110 for drying, and 129 for general information).

HORSERADISH

Get beyond its looks and use it! To do so, peel it well, then grate only as much as you need for a meal. You'll be shocked by its bite, but you'll never go back to the bottled stuff. ■ For a sauce, grate it into crème fraiche, sour cream, or yogurt with a little white wine vinegar, salt, and a touch of sugar, if desired. ■ Often scallions, chives, or dill are added, especially when served with smoked fish. ■ Make a Bloody Mary with real tomato juice and give it a kick with fresh horseradish.

JERUSALEM ARTICHOKE

Not an artichoke or from Jerusalem, but a tuber native to the United States. ■ It has a good crunch (think water chestnut) and a slightly earthy flavor, and it keeps well during the winter. ■ It can be eaten raw, such as sliced in tangy salads, or cooked. It doesn't have to be peeled, but scrub it well.

JICAMA

This root vegetable is slightly sweet, a touch nutty, and very crisp. ■ Peel well with a knife, and cut the flesh any which way. Serve in salads. Grate for an alternative cole slaw with a light citrus dressing with cilantro. ■ Excellent seasoned with lime and hot chilies. ■ Cook as a substitute for fresh water chestnuts.

KALE

see Greens, Cooking

KOHLRABI

Kohlrabi is one of the less-common members of the mustard family. It has a pleasant bite, not unlike a turnip. ■ Use the bulb only, peeled, with the stems discarded. Serve it sliced, diced, or julienned in salads for crunch. ■ Peel small bulbs and simply cook in a skillet or steam and toss with butter; eat solo or combine with other veggies. ■ Try a more labor-intensive German-style preparation: hollowed, stuffed, and roasted.

LEEK

This underused member of the onion family has a subtle flavor that adds class to any dish. ■ Cut off the root and all but the lightest green part of the foliage (use the greens for stock); clean carefully between layers to remove grit. ■ Slice or cut into long strips and plunge and dress (see page 116) with a vinaigrette. ■ Halve lengthwise and braise with chicken stock and a touch of butter. ■ Slice and sauté to use for a base in a chicken or fish dish. ■ For a classic soup, simmer with potatoes in water or broth, then puree lightly (or leave chunky). Add a pat of butter, and/or a dash of cream, and/or greens or sliced fennel. For variations, add another cut-up vegetable or two during the simmer — root veggies at the beginning and quick-cooking greens at the last minute. ■ Fabulous sautéed slowly and then cooked in a tart.

LETTUCES

see Salad Greens

LEMONS AND LIMES

Lemons and limes are superb on just about anything. ■ Most Americans don't have access to local citrus because of where they live, but many people consider lemons and limes to be a worthwhile addition to a mostly local diet. ■ Try different varieties, such as key lime, Buddha's hand, Meyer lemon. ■ Preserved lemons add a distinctive flavor to Moroccan dishes.

MELONS

Two broad categories of melon are muskmelon and watermelon, each with plenty of varieties and flesh colors, but try any local melon you can get your hands on. ■ Muskmelons have netted skins like cantaloupe and smooth skins like honeydew. Slice in half, remove the seeds, section or peel, then cut. Muskmelons are ripe when slightly soft at the bottom and fragrant smelling. ■ Look for blemishless watermelons with no flat sides. Ripe watermelons give a hollow thump when slapped. ■ Melons are best served raw or with a splash of lemon or lime juice. ■ Puree into cool soups and drinks. ■ Toss watermelon in savory salads with tomatoes, feta, and fresh mint.

MUSHROOMS

Enjoy farmed and wild mushrooms of all kinds, sautéed, roasted, stewed, or marinated and grilled. ■ Try flavoring with thyme or with Asian seasonings. ■ Sauté in butter and shallots to top toasted slices of baguettes. ■ Make a thick or brothy mushroom soup. ■ Once a year in the spring, I serve sautéed wild morels and shallots with a touch of cream over fresh fettuccini. Wow!

MUSTARD

see Greens, Cooking

NECTARINES

see Peaches

OKRA

For some it's an acquired taste, but one that's worth acquiring. ■ Excellent in gumbos or Indian foods. ■ Fabulous deep fried.

ONIONS

The onion family is a broad one. Scallions (green onions) are often served raw; use both the whites and greens. Chives have a mild flavor; use like an herb. Shallots flavor anything with their gentle, sophisticated taste; serve with butter and wine for an instant touch of France, or use raw in salad dressings. (See also Leek.) ■ Don't underestimate the power of onions — in all varieties — to transform food. ■ Sauté until translucent to start out a soup, stew, or sauté dish. ■ Slowly sauté onions with butter until nutty brown and caramelized, then top a pizza, burger, or tart. ■ Large onions like Walla Walla and Ailsa Craig are generally the sweetest; they're excellent served raw, sliced and tossed in a salad or on grass-fed burgers. ■ I adore pickled sweet red or white onions; they're great for salads, sandwiches, and antipastos. To make them, throw sliced sweet onions into boiling water. Immediately drain, then add to a jar filled with equal parts water and white wine vinegar with sugar and salt to taste.

ORANGES, GRAPEFRUITS, AND THEIR FAMILY

Try all varieties, including blood oranges, pink grapefruits, tangelos, and clementines. To section or slice: use a knife to peel the skin and white pith, then slice across the "equator" of the fruit or insert a knife between sections, leaving the membrane behind. ■ Fabulous in tangy green salads or fruit salads, and in savory sauces, especially with fish or poultry. ■ For dessert, make a simple sorbet or food processor granita. Easier yet, serve oranges with a touch of orange liquor and grated chocolate, solo or atop local ice cream. ■ Serve fresh local grapefruits, halved, for breakfast. ■ And nothing beats a glass of fresh-squeezed juice.

PARSNIPS

Peel and cut thick slices of this sweet, earthy root vegetable into Grandma's chicken soup with dill. ■ Simmer it in a touch of water or broth with potatoes, then puree or mash (or add celery root and leeks or garlic). Add more broth, and a touch of butter or cream, if you like, for a white winter soup. ■ Grate into potato pancakes to give them a slightly sweet edge.

PEACHES AND NECTARINES

Eat these during their small window of perfection, when they are fragrant and yield slightly to the touch. ■ Peaches come in freestone varieties, with pits that easily fall way from the flesh, and clingstone varieties, where the flesh clings to the pit. Cultivars and colors vary; the white peach, for instance, has less acidity. ■ You can peel a fuzzy peach by plunging it into boiling water briefly, then into ice water. ■ Classic preparations include pies, crisps, cobblers, ice cream, jam, and chutney. ■ Split, stuff, and bake as you would a pear (see Pears). ■ With a smooth skin and firmer flesh, nectarines can have more of a bite. Use as you would peaches.

PEARS

Pears ripen after harvest and have a relatively small window when they're ready to eat. So watch them carefully, wait for the top to yield slightly to the touch, and then pounce. ■ Try all varieties, including sweet little Seckel pears. ■ Serve with any local cheese, particularly any in the blue cheese family, or in a classic fall salad with lively greens and local nuts. ■ For dessert, try poached pears, which keep well in the fridge. Peel, core, and immerse in local wine or cider and water, well sweetened and seasoned with spices (or not), then simmer until fork-tender. ■ Halve, hollow, and bake pears stuffed with a combination of their meaty centers, crushed almond or ginger cookies, local nuts, your favorite sweetener to taste, an egg to bind, and a touch of butter on top. ■ And don't forget tarts, especially pear tarte tatin. ■ Asian pears are ripe at harvest and firm to the touch; they keep well in the fridge. They have a great crunch and can be grated or sliced into salads or served with dips.

PEAS, SNOW PEAS, AND SUGAR SNAPS

Peas are best eaten soon after picking to take advantage of their gentle, sweet flavor. ■ At least once each season, take the time to shell and steam fresh peas very briefly to serve with butter. ■ Or get ambitious and make a pureed fresh pea soup (simmer peas, then puree). ■ Throw fresh peas into local bacon-seasoned risotto during the last few minutes of cooking.

For sugar snaps and snow peas, pull off their strings, from one end to the other. Then use the plunge or plunge-and-dress techniques (see page 116), taking no more than 30 seconds to cook them. I like my garden sugar snaps this way, tossed in a tiny drizzle of fresh sesame oil plus salt and hot chili pepper flakes. ■ Stir fry with other veggies. ■ Pea shoots can be found in some markets featuring Asian produce. Treat them as you would greens — delicious!

PEPPERS

Popular sweet red, orange, or yellow bell peppers are really just different varieties of ripe green peppers. ■ Eat them raw in salads. ■ Roast whole on the grill or broiler until charred, then cover until cool enough to easily peel, seed, and stem. These also freeze well. Serve them as an appetizer or puree into a sauce or soup. ■ Cook sliced peppers with onions and pile onto local sausages and buns for an upscale hot dog. ■ Green bell peppers are best served cooked and are the secret ingredient in many stewed dishes. ■ All bell peppers are tasty when stuffed and baked.

Chili peppers come in 200 varieties — many shapes, sizes, colors, and flavors. Generally the smaller the pepper, the hotter it is. ■ Slice chili peppers lengthwise and remove the seeds and membranes, the sources of their fire. Wear latex gloves or wash your hands afterward. Serve chopped or finely minced, sautéed, stewed, or raw. Add to taste as hotness varies even within the same variety. ■ All peppers are fabulous in bean dishes and stir-fries.

PERSIMMON

This fruit has a creamy texture, red-orange skin and flesh, and a tangy sweet flavor. ■ Good raw or cooked, depending on the variety.

POMEGRANATE

Split open and eat the pomegranate-colored pulp surrounding each seed. ■ Colorful in salads. ■ Use the juice for sauce, sorbet, and more.

POTATOES

One of the most versatile veggies, potatoes have a distinctive flavor yet enjoy almost any seasoning or style of cooking: frying, steaming, roasting, or baking. ■ Cook whole potatoes on the grill when you've finished grilling everything else. ■ Make fritters or oven fries. ■ Roast whole potatoes and stuff. ■ Use the toss-and-roast technique (see page 117) to cook them solo or with other vegetables, as in Roasted Harvest Vegetables (see page 125). ■ Don't overlook heirloom potatoes; you may be surprised by their unique shapes, colors, flavors, and textures.

RADISHES

One of the first vegetables to be pulled from the garden in the spring, radishes are great rolled in soft butter then dipped in salt. ■ They're good sliced in salads and sandwiches or cooked into stir-fries. ■ Flavor and bite vary greatly by variety.

RHUBARB

Tart rhubarb makes an excellent dessert. Slice stalks, peeling any large tough ones, and stew with a sweetener to taste (making sure it still has some bite). Serve this compote with yogurt, whipped cream, or ice cream. ■ Make a superb crisp or pie with or without their classic pairing of strawberries. ■ Try rhubarb mousse or fool.

RUTABAGA

see Turnips

SALAD GREENS

Flavors range broadly from gentle mâche to peppery arugula, and textures include frilly frisee, slender mizuna, and tender oak leaf lettuce. ■ Baby cooking greens, like beet and mustard greens, can be thrown into salads as well. (See also Chicory.) ■ Lettuce varieties are generally divided into crisp head, such as iceberg; butterhead, such as Boston; Romaine, commonly used in Caesar salads; and leaf lettuce. Full-flavored leaf lettuces come in infinite varieties to use solo or mixed in mesclun salads; small leaves are often prewashed. ■ Bold lettuce varieties, tangy or bitter, hold up to strong dressings and/or a warm dressing to slightly wilt them. They are also good with contrasting sweet fruit or salty cheeses. Buy a mix or taste each variety to learn what you like, then create your own mix — mild, tangy, or a combination. Throw fragile herb leaves such as chervil or parsley into these salad mixes, too! ■ Always thoroughly wash and dry lettuce; salad spinners are a great time saver. ■ Toss in a dressing at the last minute, just to coat (see page 118).

SALSIFY

This long root vegetable generally has a white flesh under grayish skin, but also comes in other varieties. Its gentle flavor has been compared with oysters and asparagus. ■ Serve cooked as a solo vegetable or in soups and stews.

SHALLOTS

see Onions

STRAWBERRIES

A short local season, so eat them until you burst! If any make it home from picking, you can remove (hull) the tops, split the berries, and toss in sugar (if needed) to bleed the juices for a few minutes, then serve with whipped cream, cream, ice cream, or strawberry shortcake (see page 127). ■ Toss sliced strawberries in a touch of sugar and a small drizzle of balsamic — delicious. ■ Make parfaits, ice cream, granita, or sorbet. ■ Blend into a frappe or strawberry daiquiri. ■ Make a classic strawberry rhubarb pie or crisp. ■ Look for tiny wild strawberries, too.

SUMMER SQUASH

see Zucchini

SWEET POTATOES OR YAMS

We generally eat sweet potatoes in this country — which are somewhat varied in flavor, texture, and taste — not yams, although their names are used interchangeably. ■ Pierce each potato a few times and bake whole to keep on hand for a perfect meal as-is or with butter — no need for sweet embellishments. ■ Contrast their sweetness with a little kick: cut into fries, skin and all, toss with good chili powder and cumin, then bake in one layer at 425°F until crisp; salt lightly and eat immediately. ■ Peel, steam, or simmer, and mash as you would potatoes. ■ To warm a winter night, make a stew of sweet potatoes with chicken or mushrooms. ■ For an African touch, make a pureed soup with peanuts. ■ And don't forget sweet potato pie.

TOMATILLOS

Sometimes called a Mexican green tomato, tomatillos are a round, green fruit with a papery husk. Their unique flavor has a slightly herbal lemony kick. ■ Remove their husks and make a fabulous pureed salsa (raw or cooked) using a touch of garlic, onion, cilantro, chili pepper, and salt to taste. (I sometimes add a pinch of sugar to balance the acid.) To cook tomatillos before adding to the salsa, simmer in water until soft, or broil or grill until slightly browned. Chill salsa for use with tortilla chips, or serve warm with beans or meat.

TOMATOES

When at their seasonal peak, fresh local tomatoes can be heaven on earth. Their sweet-acid flavor is an ideal catalyst for many kinds of dishes, but also stands alone. In most parts of the country, their peak local season is short, so use them in everything while you can — classic salads with mozzarella and basil, tomato-basil sandwiches (my favorite), Italian bread soup, or simply with olive oil, salt, and nothing else. Chop them into salsas with basil or cilantro and some onion, garlic, and hot peppers. (You'll never eat the bottled stuff again.) ■ Buy or grow the endless varieties of heirloom tomatoes in all sizes, shapes, colors, and flavors.

TURNIPS AND RUTABAGAS

Peel all but very small, tender turnips, which are surprisingly mild but have a bite much like their relative the radish. ■ Cut small turnips into similar-size pieces and caramelize them by tossing them with oil and salt, then roasting at 400–450°F until browned and tender. ■ Throw large or small pieces into vegetable or meat stews. ■ Rutabagas, also called Swedes, are thought to be a cross between a cabbage and a turnip; they're larger than a turnip and are often purple at the top. Choose those that are heavy for their size and cook as you would turnips. ■ Serve in layers in a classic gratin with potatoes and cream, or mash with potatoes.

WATERMELON

see Melons

WINTER SQUASH

Hearty winter squashes include acorn, butternut, carnival, delicata, hubbard (great for pie), turban, spaghetti (with a white spaghetti-like flesh), and many others. They may vary in texture, size, and flavor, but most respond well to similar preparations: whole or split, then seeded, peeled, and cubed if needed. ■ Split and steam or roast until soft, then remove the seeds. Serve right in the skin, or scrape the flesh and mash it. When serving mashed, I cook squash whole to avoid messy and difficult splitting. Just pierce a few times and cook in a 400°F oven until quite soft. ■ Squash needs surprisingly little seasoning, although butter, maple syrup, and spices like cinnamon are favorites. Try also butter, salt, and pepper with a tiny kick of ginger or a touch of aromatic sage. ■ Use pureed sugar pumpkin — or my favorite, hubbard — for superb pie, draining well before baking. ■ Peel and cube larger squash like butternut. I like cubes cooked in grass-fed beef and bean chili, or any meat or veggie soup or stew. Kids like cubes tossed with butter, maple syrup, and spices then baked until brown in the oven. ■ For another treat, hollow a sugar pumpkin, scrape it out well, fill it with chopped apples and pumpkin pie spices, dried fruit, and a touch of cider and/or brandy. Bake it whole and serve the filling with cooked pumpkin and local ice cream.

ZUCCHINI AND OTHER SOFT-SKINNED SUMMER SQUASH

I've lumped soft summer squashes here, with zucchini (my favorite) in a starring role. All can be cooked similarly, including the common summer squash, which is yellow. Patty pan is a round variety and should be treated gently (steamed) when young. ■ Summer squash, including zucchini, need not be boring. Although it's best at about 6 inches long, it can be cooked at any size. ■ Slice and sauté over high heat in olive oil, shaking the pan to partly brown the squash and intensify the flavor; sprinkle with salt, hot chili pepper flakes, and a tiny touch of Parmesan. ■ Slice or julienne, batter lightly with a flour and water mixture, then pan fry, drain, and sprinkle with salt. Serve with a lemon wedge. (Do the same for the blossom.) ■ Slice lengthwise, toss in oil, then grill alone or with other summer veggies. ■ Steam and toss with fresh herbs and butter for a gentle flavor. ■ Layer slices in casseroles or in a vegetable Napoleon with other summer fare, like roasted eggplant, tomatoes, fresh local cheeses, and so on.

Other Local Ingredients

More information about key local ingredients will help you make smart decisions that are right for you. As you can see, issues of local food and sustainability mix quite freely here, and for good reason.

ALCOHOLIC BEVERAGES

Wine. Drinking wines crafted with regional grapes from small-scale producers is one of the easiest ways to enjoy locally grown food. While California is still the principle American source for wine, other regions have excellent selections, too, especially New York and Oregon. Look on the label for wines that use regional grapes, bearing in mind that wineries may bottle their own grapes (called estate wines), buy in grapes, or do both. Buy directly from the vineyard or winery, or go to a wine shop that focuses on customer service and ask what's local and sustainable. Most vineyards at least use IPM (see glossary). Others go further with organic or biodynamic methods. This country is still discovering its wine identity, and the combination of nascent wine traditions and rugged individualism make for flavors that are very producer-driven, so taste around.

Beer. You won't find traditional beer made with local ingredients everywhere, because its principal ingredient, barley, is primarily grown in the Midwest. Another main ingredient, hops, is mostly grown in the Pacific Northwest. There are exceptions, of course, but your beer label (or bartender) will let you know if the grain is grown locally, or you can call the brewer and find out. Bear in mind that, as with wine, the location where the beer is processed is not necessarily where its ingredients were grown. But if you can't find beer with regional ingredients, consider drinking regional microbrewed beers as a way to support local businesses and save the gas it takes to ship the heavy liquid around the country. If you can't buy directly from the brewery, look for local beers at liquor stores, specialty food stores, and restaurants.

Other beverages. You can turn almost anything into an alcoholic drink. Some excellent (and some terrible) alcoholic drinks are made from locally grown products — and you can expect more to come, as distilleries pop up all over the country. Try those using local apples, like sparkling cider, which can be heavenly. But don't limit yourself. Experiment and use local alcoholic beverages in your cooking, as well.

AMERICANS ADORE SHRIMP

The vast majority of shrimp consumed in the United States is imported from Asia and South America and is industrially farm raised. Farm-raised U.S. shrimp is an accepted ecofriendly choice, though it can be a challenge to find. Regional wild shrimp are available from the southeast Atlantic coast and the Gulf of Mexico, Maine pink shrimp are sold in the winter, and trap-caught spot prawns are found on the West Coast.

DAIRY

see Raw Milk on page 68

EGGS

Local eggs are much fresher and usually have their farm name right on the carton. But if you are looking for local and sustainably raised eggs, here are some tips. Don't favor brown over white, as color is determined by genetics and is not an indicator of taste. (My local farmer sells multicolored eggs.) When possible, buy eggs from small, sustainable farms. Local organic certified or certified humane (raised and handled like organic with less regulation on feed) are good choices, but often the carton says neither. (Mine don't.) When in doubt, find out from your vendor or farm how the chickens were raised. Many farms, like Crazy Wife around the corner from me, raise their chickens on good local grain and feed them well, but are not organic. At the very least, you want eggs from chickens that were raised without antibiotics or hormones. Bear in mind that "cage-free" chickens in large factory farms aren't strutting about joyously in the sun, but are most likely crammed together. (Look for "pasture-raised" instead.) If you wonder why you should bother with fresh local eggs at all, there's plenty written about those vile chicken farms — ugh!

Bear in mind that less than one percent of the fish entering the United States is inspected. Federally mandated COOL (country of origin labeling) will at least tell you if your fish is from this country.

FRESHWATER FISH

There are plenty of quality freshwater fish in the rivers and lakes of this country. Ask your purveyor about regional fresh fish, or try fishing with a friend. Find out where your fish comes from, as some bodies of water are too polluted to be a good food source.

FISH AND SEAFOOD

Eat local fish when you can, but consider the ethical issues when you do so. We don't want to contribute to the ocean's destruction by eating fish caught or raised without standards. So, as with sustainable cooking, try to be flexible and make substitutions when you can't buy what you want, bearing in mind that, like produce, ocean fare is seasonal.

Luckily, you can at least begin to buy with both locality and ecology in mind by checking regional watch lists. These lists outline what seafood is available regionally, sorted into what you can enjoy, should avoid, or can use for substitutions. Note that *available* doesn't always mean *regional*, so you'll have to ask. Here are three good questions to ask before buying seafood: Do you know where this seafood comes from? Do you know if it's farmed or wild-caught? If it's wild, how was it caught?

The Monterey Bay Aquarium is an excellent resource for more information about ecofriendly fish consumption. Their Web site (see Resources) provides downloadable, pocket-sized, regional lists (as well as a list for seafood used in sushi), a searchable database, recommendations on what to buy, and more information about your favorite seafood items. Once you have the hang of what's local, you can instantly find out what's sustainable by using FishPhone, The Blue Ocean Institute's sustainable seafood text messaging service. Just text 30644 with the message FISH and the name

KEEP IT COLD, GET IT FRESH

Buy regional fish and seafood very fresh, keep it very cold — I set wrapped fish over an ice cube tray or bowl of ice — and cook it as soon as possible after buying it. Patronize sources that can answer your questions about origins, know what day the catch arrives, and move fish quickly.

Seek Out Distinctive, Regional Heirloom Grains Near You

Glenn Roberts, owner of Anson Mills, in Columbia, South Carolina, grows, harvests, and mills nearly extinct varieties of heirloom corn, rice, and wheat, recreating ingredients that were in the Southern larder before the Civil War. Grits, cornmeal, Carolina Gold rice, and graham and biscuit flour, milled fresh for the table daily, have revived a celebrated regional cuisine.

Anson Mills also provides grants for growers to plant antebellum varieties of corn, and offers them heirloom seed, seed selection expertise, and management advice. To date, Roberts, who made this a personal mission when he found he couldn't create dishes from his mother's youth, now works with 30 organic growers in six states, seeking those who can make peace with the lower yields and higher demands of heirloom grains. He describes freshly ground grain as radically different, with "a huge nuttiness and flavor, almost a floral-mineral component."

---

of the fish in question, and they'll text back an assessment and better alternatives to fish that have significant environmental concerns.

Consider buying your favorite restaurant a copy of *Seafood Solutions*, a guide for chefs on buying sustainable seafood from the Chefs Collaborative. And if you want to dig deeper, visit The Blue Ocean Institute for extensive buying resources, ocean conservation, and much more. Also read *Bottomfeeder: How to Eat Ethically in a World of Vanishing Seafood* by Taras Grescoe.

GRAINS

Though hardly the norm, local grain and grain mills are slowly emerging across the country and are worth tracking down. The Midwest and northern plains may be the grain belt, but smaller pockets of grain are grown almost everywhere. Most grain, especially the bulk of the U.S. crop — corn, wheat, and rice — is grown industrially and distributed both nationally and globally. It is also sometimes genetically modified (see Glossary). Other grains grown in the United States include spelt (a relative of wheat), millet, rye, barley, and pseudograins amaranth and buckwheat.

Find local grains in green markets, small retail stores, or gourmet shops, or ask a farmer who raises animals where they're getting grain, then connect with a purveyor who might grow grain for human consumption. Remember, if you buy it whole, you are going to have to buy a home grinder. Or ask a local baker making quality bread if he or she buys grain from a small, regional mill.

To process whole grains yourself, use a home mill, grinding from frozen grain. To store, keep milled grain well sealed and always as cold as possible (the freezer is best, fridge second best, cold pantry or secure spot in the cellar third).

Wild rice is not really rice, but a long-grain marsh grass native to America. It is generally harvested by hand in the Great Lakes area, especially Minnesota and Wisconsin, by local Native Americans. Theirs is a truly sustainable method, leaving behind plenty of seed to sow next year's harvest. Commercially cultivated paddy rice is available in areas such as California and the Midwest. Other varieties of local wild rice are available along the Atlantic and Gulf Coasts, as well as in Texas.

MEAT AND POULTRY

With the consolidation of the industry, local meat, and often even poultry, is still the exception, not the rule. So if you find it, it's likely to be labeled with the name and sometimes the location of the farm. And there's probably a real person to ask — farmer or

WHERE'S MY MEAT COMING FROM?

If you are looking for more assurances, the key, once again, is to know your farmer, butcher, or retail vendor. Labels help sometimes, but not always. Local, organic certified meats may be labeled as such, but not always; organic poultry is more readily available but often not local. "All natural" doesn't tell you much. According to the USDA, all-natural meat has been "minimally processed and contains no artificial ingredients," but it does not prohibit growth hormones and antibiotics; it has to say so to be so. Some labels may indicate humane treatment of animals (with terms like "certified humane" or "cage-free"), but, as ever, it's important to know your source. So ask, ask, ask, and follow my advice!

What's the Story with Grass?

Pasture-raised meat comes from animals like cattle, buffalo, goats, sheep, and poultry that grazed on grass, their natural feed. It's a more humane and ecological method; their manure feeds the grass that in turn feeds them. Note that pigs are not usually solely pasture raised, since they need a high proportion of grain in their diet. Poultry is usually fed at least some grain.

As defined by the American Grassfed Association, grass-fed animals are fed grass and hay exclusively, except for their mothers' milk. This includes dairy animals, too. Sometimes this process is called "grass fed and finished." The term "pasture finished" enters a gray area. Those animals may be fed on grass only or have spent some or even most of their life on grass. You may see these animals referred to as "grass fed and grain finished." Ask the farmer, as the terms are sometimes loosely used and no industry standard currently exists.

All animals that are raised primarily on grass, but especially those that are solely grass-fed, produce meat that is lower in saturated fats and calories, higher in essential nutrients. Grass-fed meat also has a more distinctive flavor than factory-farmed, grain-fed meat. The full, minerally flavor of grass-fed meat is loved by many, but can be an acquired taste for some. Americans are used to grain-fed meat, which is more marbled with fat throughout and has a buttery, less meaty flavor. Unless well-raised and cooked properly, grass-fed meat can be less tender than we are used to. But you will notice that all meat from the farm is more flavorful than factory-raised meat. And it's fresh, "clean" meat!

Why doesn't every farmer pasture-raise meats? After all, these animals are raised in a more humane environment for both farmers and their animals and in a manner less destructive to the planet. One of many reasons is that grass-fed animals fatten slowly, lengthening the time it takes from birth to market. Another is that it's easiest to raise thousands of cows in a confined area.

Pasture-raised meat is seasonal, growing best when the grazing is best. In New England, I put in my order in the early spring and receive my meat in the late fall.

retailer — about how it was raised. Look for local farms with less than 1,000 animals, which are more likely to raise their livestock in a more environmentally responsive and humane manner, although some larger "boutique" farmers do so as well.

The Best Choice

The best choice is local meat and poultry from pasture-raised animals that are not raised on huge factory farms. Local certified organic meat is great, but it can be hard to find, since it's expensive to raise animals this way. Sustainably raised animals fed on pasture are generally easier to find.

But what does sustainably raised mean? The definition is open to debate, but I think it is fair to say that these are animals raised at least partly, if not entirely, on grass and that any grain used is local, sustainably grown when possible. It also means that no growth hormones are ever used and that antibiotics are used only when essential, which should be infrequently in a healthy herd. And finally, it means that both animals and workers are treated humanely. Fortunately, these practices are becoming more common on smaller farms.

How Do I Cook It?

For red meat, cook tender cuts rare or medium rare; less tender cuts, like chuck, should be cooked at a very low temperature in a slow oven or on a stovetop, covered, with some liquid for moisture.

Cook fresh, local poultry as you would conventionally raised poultry, bearing in mind that it may have less fat, so it may need a bit more liquid or basting while it cooks. The difference in flavor will astonish you.

CHANGE THE RULES

Interested in changing current regulations that make it hard for small farmers to grow and process meat? Look at the policy section on page 202.

Healthy Meat from Happy Pigs

"What my customers like best is knowing that every animal is raised on my place, from birth to death, and I am a one-man army, controlling all their inputs while treating them humanely. The only danger here is the traffic from people stopping to watch my pigs running around the farm."

BOB KITCHEN

Pigasso Farm, Copake, New York

The Cost

Sustainably raised meat and poultry can be more expensive, but the benefits are worth it and the cost can be mitigated simply by eating less of it. Not a bad idea, considering that Americans eat an average of half a pound of meat per day!

Why Bother?

I've focused on the procurement, flavor, and preparation of sustainably raised meats. But many have waxed poetic about the need to support alternatives to conventional factory farms, which are inhumane to workers and animals, marginally safe, energy-guzzling, and crammed with animals that are grown on corn (unnatural to their diet), pumped up on hormones, and fed antibiotics to cope with their disease-prone feedlots. These major polluters of land, water, and air are consolidated into the hands of a few companies. Get the picture? The pleasure of eating "clean" meat and poultry is not only in its flavor, but also its meaning.

To follow one feedlot steer's life, hoof to plate, read Michael Pollan's article *Power Steer* in the March 31, 2002, edition of *The New York Times*.

Where to Find It?

It isn't always easy to find it, but sustainably raised meat can be bought at farmers' markets, farm stands, some retailers and co-ops, specialty stores, directly from farms, and through buying clubs, also called meat CSAs (see page 48). Larger chains often stock "natural" meats from far afield but rarely local meats.

POULTRY

see Meat and Poultry

PRODUCE

Farmers tell me that, along with "What do I do with it?" the most common market question is "How long does it last?" The answer depends on

BUY FUNKY FRUIT, STRANGELY SHAPED TOMATOES, AND OTHER ALIEN PRODUCE

Don't be scared off if items look different from what you're used to. The multi-lobed, irregularly shaped heirloom tomatoes you find at a farmers' market — the ones that are hard to cut up evenly — may be the best tomatoes you've ever tried.

how fresh the produce was when you bought it, on what it is (tiny greens or an unripe pear), and how you store it. While local produce can be especially fresh, lasting a week (or more) in the fridge, it generally tastes best when eaten fairly quickly after you buy it. Just do your best and enjoy. If something looks fragile, like raspberries, it won't last long. Sturdy veggies, like cabbage, are great keepers. Use those fragile ingredients first, leaving the rest for later. Items that have been damaged in any way spoil quickly, so eat them or cook them first. Don't be afraid to leave slightly unripe tomatoes, pears, and other fruits out to ripen. If in doubt, here's the mantra again: ask. But also trust your eyes, nose, and palate.

How Do I Store It?

For the crazy clean washers among you: don't wash produce until you are ready to use it, because moisture can damage it while it's being stored. The sooner it's eaten after it's cut, the better, although when pushed, I occasionally prep vegetables a day before using.

Of course most, but not all, produce should be chilled to keep it fresh. (Remember, it's alive when you buy it and chilling retards its demise.) In the best of possible worlds, keep peppers, eggplants, cucumbers, and fully ripened melons in the fridge no more than three to four days. For storage, reuse plastic bags, as well as resealable plastic and glass containers.

Keep broccoli and cauliflower tightly wrapped in the crisper drawer. Lettuce should be tightly wrapped, unwashed. Cooking greens are especially fragile and are best cooked quickly after purchasing, but can be kept in plastic with a paper towel to absorb moisture. Store asparagus in the fridge in an upright container, like a glass or pitcher, with the ends in water and tops covered by a moist paper towel or plastic bag. Mushrooms like to be dry, so put them in an open container, such as a small colander. Corn should be stored in its husk to keep it moist. Keep eggplants in the crisper drawer of your fridge with a paper towel to absorb moisture. Zucchini and summer (yellow) squash are perishable; wrap them well and use them quickly. Cherries keep well for a week (or even two) in a tight plastic bag. Cabbage and brussels sprouts store a while in the fridge. Green beans will keep tightly wrapped in a crisper drawer.

Some produce shouldn't be chilled. Don't refrigerate potatoes, sweet potatoes, garlic, and onions; store them in a cool, dark place, if possible, to prevent sprouting. (Leeks and green onions are in the onion family but should be chilled.) Never chill a tomato because it loses its taste and texture. If it gets too ripe, cook it. You don't have to chill winter squash either, although they like to be kept cool. Lemons and limes are best kept out of the fridge. Strawberries and raspberries are best eaten unchilled when you arrive home, but they fade fast, so they have to be chilled if you plan to keep them. In fact, icy cold dulls the flavor of all fruit (and most food), so when planning to serve fruit that's been chilled, take it out of the fridge just a bit before eating.

For storing garlic and herbs, see pages 107, 109, and 110. For storing root vegetables over the winter, see page 107.

What If I Buy Too Much and Things Start to Go Bad?

Cut off anything awful and cook what's left. If it's still too lousy, compost it!

SWEETENERS: MAPLE SYRUP AND HONEY

Honey and maple syrup are great local alternatives to sugar. Maple syrup is produced in northern climates, mostly Canada and the United States, by reducing sap to syrup by boiling off the water. (One local codger told me that when she was young, they boiled it "until the wallpaper starts to peel.")

Traditionally, maple syrup is produced in a sugar house (or shack), during sugaring season in the late winter–early spring, when the freezing nights are followed by daytime temperatures that rise above 40°F. Tapping for maple sap, however, is generally done only in the spring when the weather is more predictable and the sap's sugar content is high. (The proportion of sap to syrup runs around 40 to 1.)

When shopping, carefully read labels, looking for local or regional farm locations. Quite often, even here in maple country, stores stock syrup from far away even when syrup is being manufactured close by. Some farms sell right off their property. If you have a chance, be sure to visit one during the season. (Mine, Ioka Valley Farm, sells pancakes, too.) Or tap your own maple trees to make syrup with simple equipment bought at your hardware store or online. Maple syrup comes in two grades: try both the lighter A grade and the less expensive, more maple-flavored B. If there are no maple trees near you, there's no local maple syrup. Try honey or jam, or grow and dry stevia for sweetening.

Honey is produced by bees from nectar collected from cultivated and wild flowers. It has long been a favorite for its distinctive flavor and health benefits. Honey's flavor varies greatly and depends on what the bees pollinate. Clover and alfalfa yield a mild, light-colored honey and buckwheat and wildflower honeys are darker with a stronger taste.

Local availability varies, but honey is sold in a number of ways: comb honey (stored in beeswax combs by bees), liquid honey (extracted), chunk honey (comb with liquid), and granulated honey (creamed and spreadable).

Sadly, nature's pollinators, our favorite insect farmers, are disappearing. But, it's possible to become a beekeeper almost anywhere, like Peter Hoffman, chef-owner of Savoy in New York City, who keeps hives on the roof of his apartment building.

Honey keeps forever. Store it in a cool place away from direct sunlight, but not in the fridge, because the low temperature makes it hard to pour. If it gets cloudy, it is just crystallizing, which is not harmful (I like it); reliquefy the honey by heating it gently.

The best places to find local honey are farm stands, farms, and sometimes co-ops, as well as specialty food stores or your local beekeeper.

WATER

Why drink the purified water from international beverage companies when you can drink local water? I'm lucky enough to have good well water, but if you are already buying water, switch to something from local or regional sources. If it's hard to find, stock up when you do locate it.

WINE

see Alcoholic Beverages

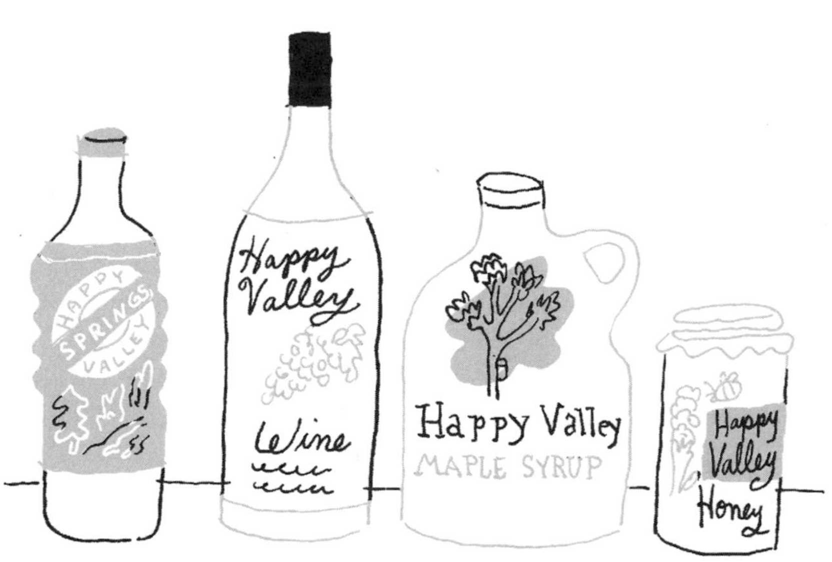

STEP THREE

CONNECT AND ENGAGE

For the last step, ditch your old consumer self — picking stuff up, taking stuff home. Instead take the locavore way, by growing your own food. Or go one step further by building better farm-to-table connections for a healthier food system in your town, region, the world.

Rather than buying uniform raspberries, pressed like a brigade of soldiers into their clear plastic square, stain your hands with your own berries picked at peak freshness. Watch chive blossoms bloom on your city windowsill, then whirr them into dressing for your scissor-cut summer salad. Don't stand on the sidelines, but complete the soil-to-table connection yourself by digging your hands in and watching food grow.

Turn personal into political by connecting your locavore's passion to the world. For it will take all of us to heal our broken industrial food system. Imagine moving away from a nation of semis traveling cross-country loaded with "food" grown in dead soil and instead toward thriving communities growing their own vibrant food in a landscape bursting with biodiversity.

In city sills or country plots, you can harvest radically fresh food at its peak, connect with the passing seasons, wait for the sun to turn potted tomatoes ripe or for the soil to warm enough to receive seeds. After pressing peas into the ground, you can watch the pods fatten on their vine, wait anxiously until you pluck and shuck them, then savor them warm with a toss of sweet butter. Celebrate the glory of how food grows in your garden, small or large, well ordered or wild with weeds. And salute the farmers who do this for us every day.

You can be part of building this just, sustainable food system with good food for all. Start by connecting with real people about the issues nearest to your heart. It doesn't matter where — community local food feasts, CSA shares for those in need, food policy councils, or farm-to-school programs.

Everyone eats. So growing food and sharing it, while building a better world through our universal connection to our sustenance, unites rather than divides us. So together, let's get out there and engage in this last potent step.

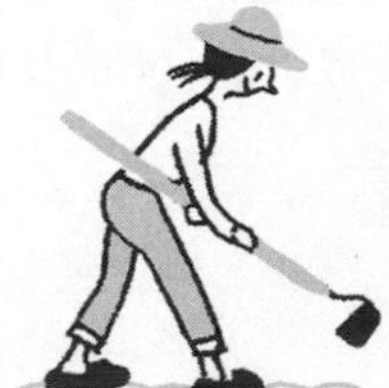

Get Your Hands Dirty

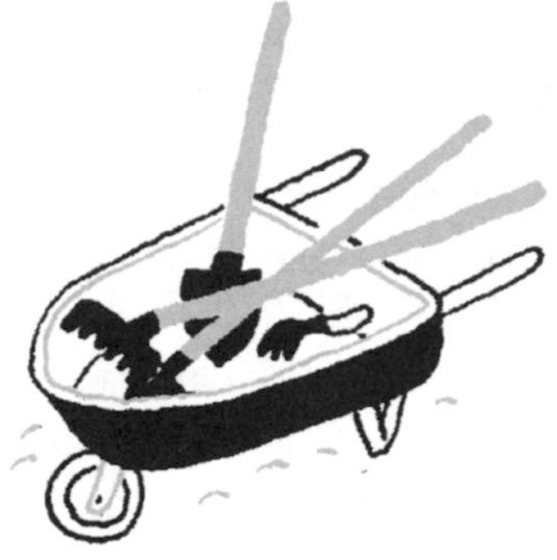

"At least in this one corner of your yard and life, you will have begun to heal the split between what you think and what you do, to commingle your identities as consumer and producer and citizen."

MICHAEL POLLAN

Food and agriculture writer

You can't get more local than food from your own backyard, windowsill, or rooftop garden. And gardening is transformative. No matter who you are, once you've picked a vegetable you've grown, you'll never feel the same about food again.

Wander out to cut salad greens for your dinner as the sun goes down. Pinch off some basil leaves to add to your sliced tomatoes. Savor the tastiest food imaginable while witnessing the miracles of nature. Watch your string beans, begun as a $2.25 bag of seeds, give birth to a festival of climbing vines, with little flowers from which tiny green bean tips emerge and then grow into something quite recognizable and savory — pounds of string beans to feed your family. Get outside and feel the rush from meaningful exercise. Become a problem solver and an active part of the food system; growing, feasting on, and sharing your own harvest.

The work you carry out in the vegetable garden will also make you a better local food shopper: you'll learn firsthand just how delicious a truly fresh vegetable is, so you won't settle for less. By gardening, you'll also gain a greater respect for farmers. (Can you imagine if you had to make a living at this?)

BECOME A KID AGAIN IN THE GARDEN

Years ago, on a chilly day before spring broke, my three-year-old daughter and I pushed holes into the soil with our fingers and dropped a shriveled pea into each. Two months later, from bushes her height, we picked sugar snap peas with a sweet pea-green flavor that was so tasty they never made it back to the kitchen.

Starting a Garden: Tips from a Lax Gardener

Here's a succinct look at vegetable gardening, which should help you decide whether you want to give it a try. If you live in the city, have no land, or want a more controlled way to garden, skip to An Alternative: Potted Crops on page 190.

WHERE'S THE VEGGIE GARDEN GOING TO GO?

Put your garden anywhere you get at least 6 hours of sun a day. You may want to site your garden near the

Symbiosis

"It is important not to isolate the components of gardening, but to see them as a whole. Everything is symbiotic: the soil, the plants, you, and the earth. Working all these things together is the key to gardening. When I started learning that, noticing the big picture, it all made sense."

JESSICA SAVORY

Senior Gardener, Berkshire Botanical Gardens, Stockbridge, Massachusetts house in order to have access to water, to remind yourself to weed, or simply to enjoy its beauty, intermingling colorful flowers with vegetables and creating pretty garden gates or fences. Also, proximity to the house (and your pet) will help to keep away animals.

WHAT SIZE?

There is no one-size-fits-all garden, but don't start too large because you're liable to create a garden that gobbles time and produces too much food. (My second garden grew wheelbarrows full of zucchini for a household of two — what was I thinking?) You can start as small as a 4-by-4-foot plot; even growing an herb or two in one pot is still satisfying. A smart gardener grows intensively, making the most of a small space, rather than taking on a huge plot that quickly gets out of control.

Another good guideline is to grow only what you can realistically handle, while keeping your garden varied enough to hold your interest. Garden plans inevitably get to be too grandiose for the slice of time you'll have to garden. Start small, including something new when you can, then expand when you feel in control.

WHAT A GARDEN NEEDS

For a good vegetable yield, all you need is healthy soil, sun, water, and sometimes a little food.

Living Soil

Soil should be alive with microorganisms, which make nutrients available for plants, one reason you don't want to add synthetic chemicals to your garden — even those that aren't designed to kill pests will destroy microbial life in the soil. Most vegetables grow well in a home of loose, well-drained, living soil that's rich in organic matter and has a pH around 6.5 (see Proper

NOURISHMENT FOR THE EYE, BODY, AND SOUL

Jessica Savory, the aptly named senior vegetable gardener at my local Berkshire Botanical Gardens, mingles her crop with cascading coral amaranth, juxtaposed with curly purple kale and light green leaves of nasturtium, punctuated with warm-colored flowers. Mixing perennial and annual flowers — some edible, others not — with contrasting vegetables adds to your gardening pleasure, boosts your salads, fills your vases, and brings around the birds. Some flowers, such as marigolds, also keep away animals and bugs.

Young Love

As a suburban kid just out of college, I dug my first garden, a 10-by-12-foot plot, next to my first rented house, a small ranch in the country. After turning the soil over with a borrowed shovel, I followed my neighbor's advice and sprinkled some lime into the soil to balance the pH, then fed it periodically with fish emulsion, a stinky gardening gift from a friend. I planted everything from seed, and it all yielded well (except for the carrots) and brought me great joy. Since then I've had gardens as large as 1,000 square feet (much too large), but I've now settled on nine 4-by-4-foot raised beds, which feel just right. Most years I plant them all, but like many gardeners, I have off years when summer work absorbs me, so I plant too little, forget to replant, or let the weeds get out of control. But even then I harvest something wonderful — a small basket of sugar snap peas, some tangy arugula, or enough tomatillos to make a batch of salsa. Besides, it's ideal to balance growing your own with visits to the CSA, farm stand, and farmers' market.

---

pH and Rotation, below). You can buy a pH testing kit at a hardware store, or you can have faith and trust your neighbors, which is what I do.

Plants need varying amounts of three major nutrients — nitrogen, phosphorus, and potassium (often represented by their chemical symbols N-P-K) — and a dizzying array of micronutrients. Although it's possible to supply the Big Three with a store-bought fertilizer, it's best to try and provide a broader spectrum of nutrients by adding generous amounts of good-quality compost to the soil. Think of it as comparable to a human being trying to eat exactly the right amounts of carbohydrates, protein, and fat, but completely ignoring whether they're getting all their vitamins. An easy way around the problem is to simply eat a wide variety of foods and trust that you're getting what you need. Adding compost to the garden once or twice a year will go a long way toward making sure your plants have all the nutrients they need.

Proper pH and Rotation

Although I know that many gardeners never test their soil and still raise robust vegetables, it is helpful to know, especially if your garden's not doing well, that most vegetables thrive in a slightly acidic soil with a pH around 6.5 (7 is neutral). In the fall or early spring, you can sweeten (raise the pH of) your soil by adding lime, or acidify (lower the pH of) your soil by adding peat moss or aged pine wood shavings.

Rotating crops from one year to the next is a good idea, to help replenish the soil and to avoid the buildup of pests and diseases that favor particular plants. For example, you wouldn't want to plant corn in the same spot every year, because it's considered a "heavy feeder" (it needs large amounts of nutrients to grow well). To offset this, you'd follow it in the next planting season with something like peas, which actually return nutrients to the soil. If each year you choose nourishing plants for areas where heavier feeders grew, you'll have happier plants all around and a better yield, too.

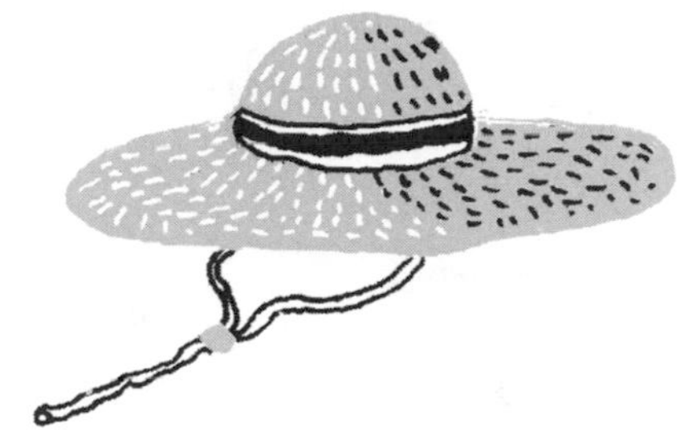

Sun

Remember photosynthesis? It's a complicated process, but basically, plants use solar power to convert the water and nutrients they take up from the soil into the energy they need to grow. To produce well, most vegetables need at least 6 hours of direct sun a day. Certain leafy greens are fine in partially shade (especially in hot climates).

Water

Always water the soil after you seed or plant. I also like to soak starter plants before planting. Throughout the growing season, some plants (like tomatoes)

THE BOTTOM LINE: IS GARDENING CHEAPER THAN BUYING LOCAL FOOD?

It depends. Gardening can be much cheaper, unless you get carried away with fancy tools, fences, and raised beds. Even if you're only paying for seeds, though, you'll have to swallow some kind of start-up fee. Fortunately, it will pay itself off by the end of the season!

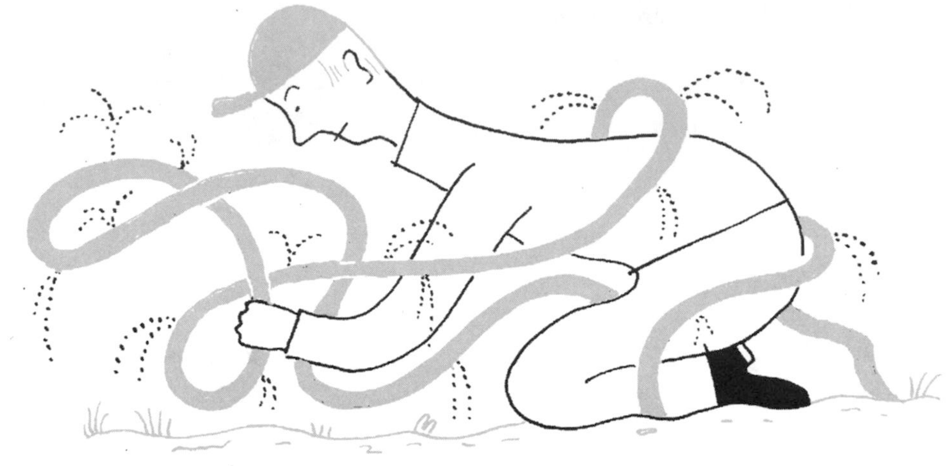

will need more water than others (rosemary), although the general rule is that gardens need an average of an inch of water a week.

To determine whether you need to water, simply poke your finger into the soil. If it isn't moist, water it. Or you can be more precise: buy a water gauge, put yourself on a watering schedule, and water when there isn't enough rain. Err on the side of more, rather than less, water and water deeply (long, slow watering rather than a quick but shallow spray from the hose) for stronger roots. You can use an irrigation system — a porous soaker hose lying on (or buried in) the garden — set on a timer or as needed. Or try a water harvesting barrel that hooks to a hose or a plastic five-gallon bucket. That's what I use.

Food

The compost you're using in your soil (see Living Soil on page 183) is already feeding your plants, but many gardeners add organic fertilizer for an extra boost during the growing season, as well. There are many options, from liquid seaweed or fish emulsion, to dehydrated cow manure.

Weeding

Weed regularly to keep unwanted plants from taking over the garden. You can simply pull them by hand; a stirrup hoe is helpful, though, especially with young weed seedlings early in the summer. Mulching with some kind of organic material such as salt hay (or whatever is available near you) helps to keep weeds at bay and decreases the evaporation of moisture from the

MAKE YOUR OWN

If you have a little extra outdoor space, consider starting your own garden compost pile out of kitchen scraps. Or if you have available basement space and are willing to be a little more selective about the scraps you save, worm composters turn leftovers into compost. Kids love watching the magic.

soil. Some gardeners plant vegetables closely together, so as to leave little room for weeds. Don't worry about being perfect. Vegetables can grow among some weeds; they just don't like to be choked by them.

Although it's good to "weed early and weed often," as the old farmers say, if you've planted seeds, wait until the seedlings are large enough for you to differentiate the weeds from the veggies. A farmer once told me, "More damage has been done by enthusiastic weeders . . ."

TOOLS

Your hands are the best tools in the garden. For the bare minimum in gardening tools, start with a shovel, a trowel, and a set of pruners (for harvesting, removing dead leaves, and trimming back plants). For no-brainer weeding, I love a stirrup hoe, which looks, well, like a stirrup. You just scrape it along the ground to cut off the weeds' tops. (If weeds get big, comfort yourself that they're easier to pull by hand.) It is also helpful, but not essential, to have a garden rake and a digging fork to spread manure and compost.

To break ground for the first time, you can either rent a rototiller or turn over your own soil by hand, using a shovel. If you're creating a garden in a lawn, be sure to slice off the sod from the area you'll be gardening before you dig in. You can either create a garden in the ground or you can build raised beds to grow in. Raised beds are mounded beds of soil, 8 to 12 inches

FOR THE LAZY LOCAVORE WITH DOUGH

Want fresh garden produce without the work? Locavores in the city, country, and suburbs — with money but no time — are paying gardeners to put in organic vegetable plots, tend them, and harvest the results.

above ground, sometimes supported by a frame. They improve drainage and help prevent soil compaction, because you walk *around* rather than *in* the beds. You can buy frames in wood or other ecofriendly materials, or you can make your own. I like them because, for lazy gardeners like me, they create a neat-looking garden. Beds can be any size, but don't make them too much wider than four feet, otherwise you won't be able to reach the middle without stepping into the bed!

TO FENCE OR NOT

If you can get away without a fence, don't bother with one. But if you need to keep animals out (like I do), a fence is essential. I wasn't happy when deer ate the leaves of my sunflowers. I was angry when they came back the next day to eat the flower heads. But I got even angrier when a family of lumbering groundhogs ate most of my vegetable crop. I asked my husband to put in a fence. (*Tales of Peter Cottontail* did not bring back my sense of humor.)

All fences are not alike, so consider what kinds of animals you need to keep out and build your fence accordingly. For example, deer fencing should be at least 8 feet high. A fence meant to keep out burrowing animals will need to be buried at least a foot belowground. Electric fences keep everything away, but they can be costly, especially if you have a large area to enclose.

GARDENING STARTS

You can plant vegetables from seeds or as starter plants. Starter plants give you a jump on the season, which is especially helpful in northern climates.

CROPS THAT TASTE BETTER STRAIGHT FROM THE GARDEN

- berries of all kinds
- broccoli
- cilantro
- cucumbers (harvested on the small side)
- green beans
- lettuces, especially lettuce mixes (mesclun)
- peas
- sugar snap peas
- tarragon
- tomatoes, especially heirlooms
- zucchini (because you can harvest them small)

PLANTING

When to Plant

Each region has its own growing season, and some regions grow food year-round. Seed catalogs are a good source for information on when to plant. They often contain charts that will tell you when to start seeds, based on where you live. The easiest way to get a garden going, though, is to buy started plants from the farmers' market and simply asking the grower for advice. If you need more help from then on, get in touch with your local cooperative extension office (see Resources).

LIVE IN THE CITY?

Community gardens are a common way for urban dwellers to grow their own vegetables. To find a community garden near you, turn to Resources.

What to Plant

That's the big question, and the start of all the fun. Once again, seed catalogs are your most up-to-date resource for ideas on what to plant. Start with the vegetables you know you like to eat. You'll also want to plant crops that will mature at different times throughout the season. (Everything in my second garden came in at once and I couldn't keep up with it.) This staggered planting will help you enjoy the garden over

---

CROPS THAT ARE WORTH PLANTING TO SAVE MONEY

- artichokes
- berries of all kinds
- edible decorative flowers, such as nasturtium, calendula, Johnny-jump-ups
- fingerling potatoes
- garlic
- heirloom or any unusual or unusually colored cultivar
- heirloom tomatoes
- herbs, because you can pick what you need
- leeks
- melons of all kinds
- mesclun mix, baby lettuces of all kinds
- perennial herbs (harvest what you need)
- shallots

the entire growing season. If you're a planner, pencil and paper help here.

It's also a good idea to plant a few surefire plants (like summer squash) with new ones. That way, you'll get some guaranteed return and, if you're lucky, some surprises, too. I tend to plant a few items that are tough to find — such as meaty Roma beans or heirloom vegetable varieties — along with herbs I like to have on hand and lots of salad greens. There are also the usual "safeties" — the easy-to-grow crops, such as cucumbers and zucchini — along with one or two new crops a season, just to break it up.

EXTENDING THE GROWING SEASON

Growing plants indoors or in a cold frame or hoop house out of season takes a bit more interest, time, and skill, but it is a superb way to prolong the season and well worth looking into. You can use simple techniques, like growing spinach in a cold frame, bringing herbs indoors to overwinter on a sunny sill, or sprouting seeds through the winter. Even in frigid Maine, Eliot Coleman and Barbara Damrosch, organic farmers and authors, grow vegetables straight through the winter. (See Recommended Reading.)

> Some perennial herbs, like rosemary, can survive indoors during the colder months and then be placed outside (or kept on a windowsill) when summer arrives.

An Alternative: Potted Crops

Growing potted plants is a way to enjoy gardening if you have limited space, hate to weed, or want more control over your garden. Growing outside is best, but if you have a very sunny south-facing window, you can grow some vegetables indoors, too.

For convenience, if possible, keep pots near a water source, as you'll be watering often. Make sure to use a very well-drained pot with holes along the bottom and/or sides. When you water, make sure the water drains out the bottom. Except for herbs, don't allow the soil to dry out completely between waterings. Plants in containers need more watering than those growing in the ground, and if the containers are in full sun, it's very likely that you'll be watering at least once a day during the summer. Alternatively, you can try gardening in self-watering containers, which provide a steady supply of water to the plants. (See the books by Ed Smith in Recommended Reading.)

"God Almighty first planted a garden: and, indeed, it is the purest of human pleasures."

FRANCIS BACON
philosopher

WHAT'S INSIDE?

For a good potting soil, combine one part planting mix (often called potting soil) and one part compost, preferably both organic. The compost will help retain water, nourish plants, moderate the pH, improve drainage, and much more. Add an organic fertilizer as needed to keep plants healthy and productive (try once a month, to start).

WHAT TO PLANT IN POTS

Some vegetables grow very well in pots, particularly those that need warmth, such as tomatoes, peppers, and eggplants. Leafy cooking greens like spinach and Swiss chard are a snap, as are radishes, which appear in no time. You're really limited only by your imagination (and the amount of sun you have, of course). Try a window box planted with herbs; add mesclun, grown from seed. Or try cucumber plants, whose vines will wander up a patio portico.

Beyond Veggies

Once you've gotten your vegetable garden off to a good start, consider planting a berry patch, keeping a goat for milk or cheese, or maybe a few chickens. Keeping hens for eggs is just one way to raise some of your own food.

FRUIT FOR YOUR YARD

Consider a fruit tree, berry bush, or rhubarb patch. Rhubarb plants came with my house, and their sweetened stewed stalks are an early harvest treat after a long winter. I put in my raspberry plants 15 years ago, and they still bear plentiful, easy-to-reach berries each year, unless I skip their early spring pruning. My daughter, Emma, grew up pushing a berry onto each finger tip, wiggling them, then eating them off each finger, one by one.

Heirloom Produce

Heirloom fruits and vegetables, especially tomatoes, have become a symbol of shockingly delicious (and often expensive) food in recent years, and they continue to gain popularity for their superb flavor. Varieties that embrace a wider spectrum of flavors and colors — yellow and orange cauliflower, blue and red potatoes, purple carrots, and a rainbow of glorious dried beans — remind us that food isn't a generic product but something to celebrate.

The term *heirloom* refers to open-pollinated produce more commonly grown during earlier times, generally 50 or more years ago, and not commonly used in contemporary agriculture. Modern varieties are bred for their durability and ability to pack and ship well. By contrast, heirlooms were bred for their distinctive flavor, although they sometimes look irregular. (When I complimented a local farmer last summer on the variety and flavor of his heirlooms, he told me that several of his farm stand clients had complained that his tomatoes were impossible to slice into perfect sandwich rounds.)

Not only are heirlooms tasty, but also when you grow or buy them, you encourage biodiversity. In the earlier part of the 20th century, we enjoyed a wide variety of each kind of vegetable. The popularity of heirloom vegetables is bringing biodiversity back into the marketplace. Only heirloom varieties "come true" from seed (meaning that they produce the same plant they came from). For information about seed saving, visit the Seed Saver's Exchange Web site (see Resources) or find a seed saver's network near you.

YOUR OWN EGGS

Raising chickens isn't for everyone, but fresh eggs, with their rich, orange, stand-up yolks, are far better than the supermarket variety, which are who-knows-how-old. And when they're connected with a story, they taste even better.

I'm lucky enough to pick up freshly laid eggs from a friend and neighbor, Ruth Dinerman, who keeps five chickens: four hens (Lucy Liu, Mandingo, Poopy Butt, and May Sarton) and one rooster named Big Red. Although she was raised in suburbia, Ruth took to the birds instantly. She claims they have different personalities — Lucy Liu is the most adventurous — and says they're selective when choosing buddies to hang out with. Big Red is sometimes aggressive, puffing himself up to protect his girls, but if you puff yourself up, too, he backs down quickly. The birds wander outside when Ruth's around, but when she's away, she puts them in their little shack or fenced area, to keep them safe from predators.

All she needed for this small egg venture was an insensitive nose, shelter from the weather (and other animals), good fencing, a few golf balls to encourage laying in some boxes or crates, and food and water provided regularly. It also helps if you don't have neighbors close by — especially if you keep a rooster. Roosters have a lot to say and no library voice.

If you can find locally raised grain, as Ruth does, you'll have eggs that are local through and through. You'll also have a steady source of chicken manure to use as a fertilizer for your garden.

How Many Eggs Do You Get?
That depends on the chicken's age, the ambient temperature, and the amount of light they receive. Another local egg farmer, Billie Best, tells me that her hens don't start laying until they're seven months old. After that, young birds can lay about an egg a day, and as they get older, they lay a few eggs a week. After they molt at about 18 months, they eventually stop laying.

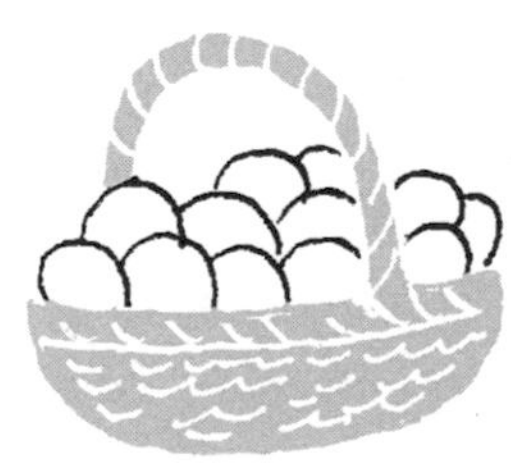

The Fiddlehead Man

Ironically I met Jack Orloff, who practices the age-old art of foraging for food, on the Internet. Other contradictions? His lumberjack frame treads lightly, so as to protect the forest undergrowth. He smokes cigarettes with one hand while foraging with the other. And, although he aims to bring fiddleheads to the front burner during their short season, he prefers to keep his real name (and prime foraging spots) secret.

Mr. Orloff, dubbed "The Fiddlehead Man" by chefs, e-mailed me when I was director of our local-food advocacy group, Berkshire Grown. He requested that I connect him with local food–friendly restaurants and stores, hoping to sell them 10-pound bags of his tasty ferns. In New England, April is a bleak time when there is scant food emerging from the earth, so I leapt at the opportunity. My stipulation? Take me foraging.

There is plenty to forage where I live in the Berkshires, and likely where you live, too. Some edible wild plants were always wild; many escaped from long-gone kitchen gardens and have since naturalized. When I first moved here, some visiting Chinese friends became giddy with the local bounty in my backyard. Fanning out, they gathered mysterious edibles that they wokked, filling the house with savory smells. Since then I've nibbled on a wild ginger root, picked numerous berries, and accepted gifts of glorious morels. But like many, I generally shy away from gathering wild foods on my own, worried about getting sick or simply too lazy to work for my dinner. But the comfort and skills of a professional forager gave me the courage to take the plunge.

As a chef, I've been familiar with fiddleheads for years, even cooked them a handful of times. Their flavor is often compared with asparagus. "Fiddlehead" is the word for all fern shoots, but it is used in the food world to refer to the young fronds of the edible ostrich fern (*Matteuccia struthiopteris*), picked before they unfurl in the spring.

BE CAREFUL

Although most wild food is not poisonous, you can't be too careful. I recommend foraging with experts, consulting books, and never taking chances. You'll find foraging groups all over the country, so connect up!

Mr. Orloff's father was a Canadian lumberjack (which explains Mr. Orloff's size) and forager who taught his son how to gather wild foods. The son considers himself a farmer, with the wilds of Massachusetts and Connecticut as his farms. He forages eight prime spots in the region, the largest is 250 acres of fiddleheads.

Once alone in the woods he explained, "Ninety-nine percent of foragers will blindfold or shoot you after they tell you their spots." Then he led me to an uneven, lower-quality spot in South County that he was willing to disclose. Generally, fiddleheads grow near water, and the setting was an idyllic workspace. A yellow finch called to its mate across the river, where Mr. Orloff pointed out more fiddleheads on the bank. They were easy to spot. In fact, once you saw one, you couldn't stop seeing the small, unfurling ferns, accompanied by larger, more mature fronds. "After I've been picking for 3 or 4 days, I see them in my dreams, even when I close my eyes," he told me.

He instructed me to walk lightly, so as not to crush the growing ferns. I could feel them underfoot, pushing up under the moist leaf-covered ground. We harvested ferns near the riverbank, picking in a circle around us, covering everything within arm's reach before moving on. We pinched off the ferns easily with our fingers, one by one. As each hand filled, we dropped the fiddleheads into five-gallon buckets, each holding up to 18 pounds when full. Simple, quiet work. The only hazards were poison ivy, deer ticks, stinging nettle, and a sore back.

The Fiddlehead Man picks about 45 pounds a day, singlehanded. His wife, swift from years of piecework at a factory, can pick up to 60 pounds in several hours. The ferns, picked with a 1- to 2-inch stem, sell wholesale to 35 regional restaurants and stores.

To prepare fiddleheads, you must clean them first by rubbing the fuzzy brown coat off with your hands and then washing them several times in cold water. Throw them into lightly salted boiling water for about 30 seconds, followed with a quick chill in ice water. Dry and sauté them in a little butter over medium heat with minced shallots until hot. Mr. Orloff says his clients have served them numerous ways — in quiches, creamy soups, even on top of pizza!

The chefs like petite fiddleheads, but The Fiddlehead Man enjoys the large ones blanched, battered, and fried, then served with a dip. On the day we picked, he had begun his foraging with a fiddlehead-sausage omelet. When I returned home with my own bag of ferns, I made myself an omelet, too. The curled, green ferns nested prettily in the yellow eggs. Their flavor held a mysterious edge from the wild, slightly exotic and woodsy, a little crisp and meaty at the stem. Their earthy flavor was tempered nicely by the creamy eggs. A spring tradition had begun.

CONSULT THE WILDMAN

The Fiddlehead Man helped me pick out edible plants. Consult *Identifying and Harvesting Edible and Medicinal Plants in Wild (and Not So Wild) Places* by Wildman Steve Brill. He teaches how to identify hundreds of edible plants, including the unfurled fiddlehead ferns, and what not to eat as well.

Become a Local Food Advocate

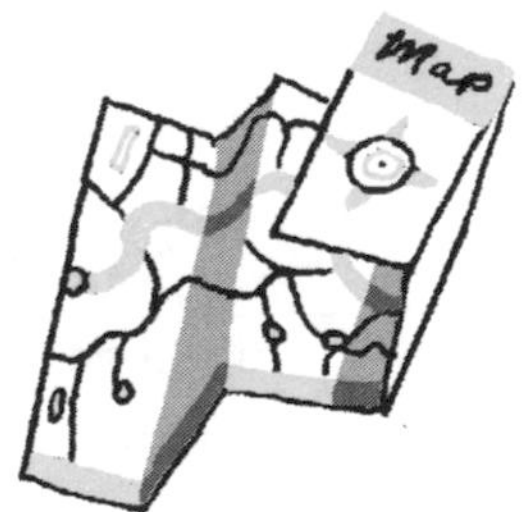

"Where are you going to be when the change occurs?"

FRED KIRSCHENMAN

Organic Farmer, Distinguished Fellow, Leopold Center for Sustainable Agriculture

You're likely to dive into the local food scene, as I did, driven by a lust for flavor, savoring it and sharing it with family and friends. But over time, eating locally came to mean something more to me — I began to see it as a way to connect with my community and the natural world, in addition to being a tangible alternative to a broken food system and offering an optimistic vision for what the future could be like. This chapter outlines some of the ways that you can help make that vision a reality.

It may not feel like you're making a difference, but shopping, savoring, and sharing local foods are all part of what Alice Water calls the Delicious Revolution that's transforming our food system, one apple at a time. Still, as a veteran farm-to-table activist, I can't help encouraging you to go one step further, making connections and engaging in your community. This chapter is a snapshot of how to do just that. It should get you jump-started, extending your local food outlook into the community to support change on a broad scale.

Participate in a way that works for you. Like exercise, you'll do it if you enjoy it. Any engagement, large or small, is one step forward. So start anywhere — by sealing envelopes, volunteering, hosting a feast of local foods, becoming a member of a local food initiative, raising money for a school garden, or developing a new local food project in your community. The list is limitless!

SUPPORT FARMERS AND FARMING

Where would we be without our farmers? Support farms, schools, and other organizations that train sustainable farmers to work in your community. It's essential if we want to localize the food system and continue to savor its bounty.

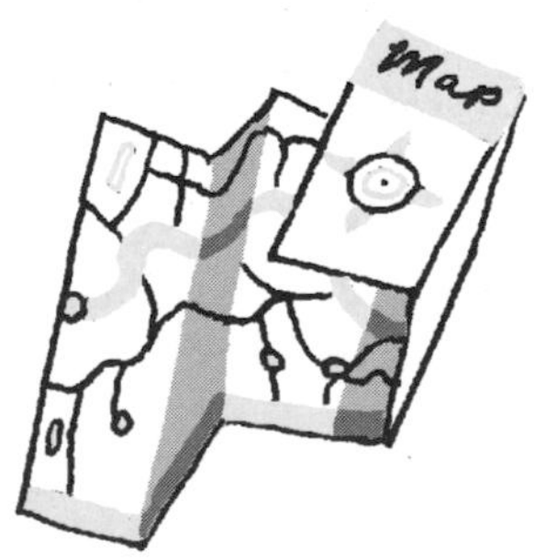

Finding Your Connection

Finding the right local connections may take a little detective work. Happily, the same sources you've discovered while learning to shop locally will help you find ways to become active in your community. Take advantage of those connections. I'll also provide you with some national and regional resources that can steer you to local, or at least regional, contacts.

START, JOIN, OR SUPPORT A LOCAL FOOD INITIATIVE

The term "local food initiative" includes everything from small groups advocating the use of local foods to regional and national nonprofits and agricultural agencies that put their training and marketing energy into supporting small and medium farms with a variety of innovative programs. It also includes groups that focus on a single project or issue, like the preservation of heritage breeds or the establishment of a community farm.

Fortunately, there are many local farm and food advocacy groups, including many buy-local campaigns. You can find or create a buy-local initiative in your region by using the Foodroutes model (see Resources) or the numerous resources throughout this book. It may also be useful to connect with a group elsewhere that you admire and ask if they know what's happening in your world.

Start by letting your passions guide you, and this will become your path to community action. (Mine is food. Ironically, it was at a conference for culinary professionals in Texas that I met Robyn Van En, Cathy Roth, and the progressive agricultural advocates who worked near me in New

No Cookie-Cutter Approach

LOCAL IS DISTINCTIVE, NOT GENERIC

My work as a farm-to-table organizer and consultant to local, regional, and national farm-to-fork initiatives has taught me that there's no single approach to reforming the food system. Initiatives work best — and certainly build the most momentum — over the long haul, when they work sustainably, through their own window into positive change, tailored to their local, often idiosyncratic, needs.

England!) Develop your own connections through your interest in the environment, health, agriculture, gardening, economic development, local economies, social justice, preserving our working landscape, and so on.

Start small and grow as needed, or connect with larger groups and you'll likely benefit from their experience and networking opportunities. Either way, my advice is to initiate and support volunteer projects where the excitement and energy are the greatest; volunteers work with their hearts as well as their heads. Look at your goals from short-term and long-term perspectives, and engage everyone in the process, even unlikely shareholders or potential opponents. (Look around: there's probably a legislator, storeowner, newspaper, or even a bank that just might join the fun.)

Finally, learn a bit about the basics of community organizing. Don't get frustrated. Only a few people do the bulk of the work. Think big, but be satisfied with small, incremental changes. You may need to set concrete projects with a beginning, middle, and end, but, if you can, think in decades, too. It takes a long time to implement change. Many helpful resources are also available online (start with the link to Sustainable Table, in Resources).

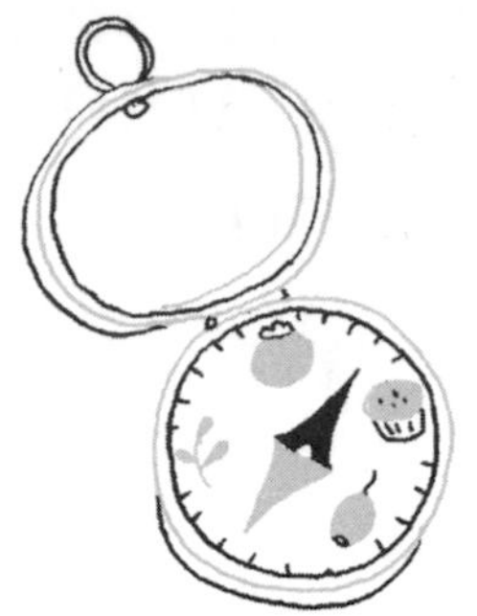

ACTIVE CULTURE

10 WAYS TO GROW YOUR LOCAL FOOD SYSTEM

Here are just a few examples of local food initiatives, large and small, which have worked well.

1 **Start an online directory of food.** Develop an online local directory or map for consumers that guides them to local food sources. (Update it regularly, and get it into the right hands.)

2 **Educate the decision makers.** Print a state-focused agricultural calendar with an educational focus, and then distribute it to all state representatives.

3 **Organize "buycotts."** Initiate or support local, state, or regional buy-local campaigns that focus on local food "buycotts" and consumer education about the importance of farms.

4 Connect farms and restaurants. Start or collaborate with farm-to-restaurant and -store networks, developed one connection at a time.

5 Preserve farmland. Support or create community land trust projects and land reserved for agriculture to preserve a diverse landscape, including the *working* landscape, like our farms (see Build a Farm-Friendly Community, page 206).

6 Support farm-product businesses. Encourage entrepreneurs and producers to access the value-added farm products with advice on production, business, and distribution.

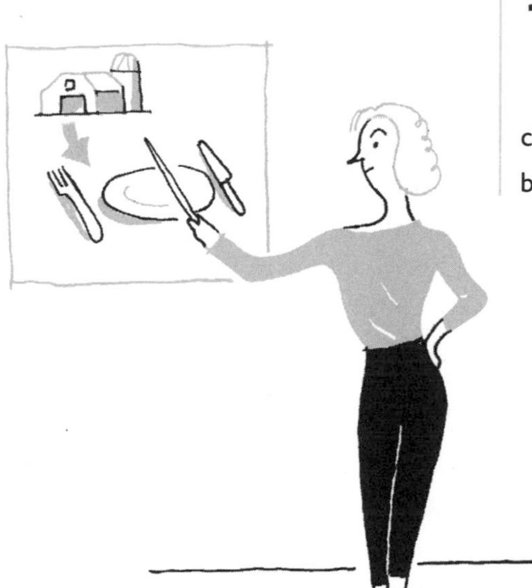

7 Start a community kitchen. Take your support of local businesses a step further and start (or help improve) a community kitchen for the development of value-added farm products.

8 Organize a bookstore promotion. Get your independent bookstores to promote independent farmers and farm advocacy groups with a weeklong promotion of books on regional foods and agriculture.

9 Start a community garden. Start or boost a community garden, enabling those who don't have land to grow their own food.

10 Arrange farm tours. Work through your food co-op and invite consumers, restaurant chefs, and others who will benefit from a behind-the-scenes look at local foods.

"Not a cup but a cow."

DAN WEST

Founder of Heifer International, referring to the organization's emphasis on developing self-reliance rather than providing short-term relief

FIGHT HUNGER WITH LOCAL FOOD DEMOCRACY

You've already read about becoming a thoughtful food consumer, which is an important task. We also need to be good food citizens, not only supporting healthy local food that's sustainably raised but making it *accessible to all*. You can address this daunting task tangibly on a local level by making sure that fresh farmers' market food is available for low-income families. Ask if your farmers' market participates in the WIC (Women, Infants, and Children) or Senior Farmers' Market Nutrition Program (SFMNP), both of which provide eligible participants with vouchers for fresh produce. A growing number of markets also now accept EBT (Electronic Benefits Transfer) from the Supplemental Nutrition Assistance Program (SNAP, formerly food stamps) through wireless point-of-sale (POS) terminals that sometimes double as credit/debit machines (ATMs). Because the costs of becoming an authorized dealer of EBT can be prohibitive for smaller farmers' markets, as of 2008, fewer than 10 percent of farmers' markets participated in the program. You can help by encouraging your market to start accepting EBT or by offering to help raise money to cover the costs of a wireless POS device. Funding for new EBT projects is also available through the USDA's Farmers Market Promotion Program

Healthy CSA food should be available for all, too. Support food banks that partner with CSAs. Let the low-income community know about CSAs that barter work for shares. Connect with or jump-start community organizations and faith-based groups that pool funds for CSA shares for low-income families or food pantry donations.

Look beyond the surface when you donate to charities, supporting those that give the poor opportunities to help themselves and provide access to healthy local foods. Heifer International, both here and around the world, does just that by helping communities obtain a sustainable source of food and income. You likely have organizations in your community that do tremendous good as well. How about volunteering to support their work or

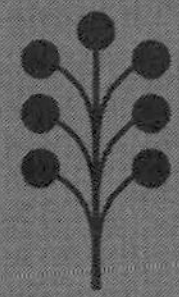

Just Food for All

"We are the food we eat, the water we drink, the air we breathe. And reclaiming democratic control over our food and water and our ecological survival is the necessary project for our freedom."

VANDANA SHIVA
Earth Democracy

"Community food security is a condition in which all community residents obtain a safe, culturally acceptable, nutritionally adequate diet through a sustainable food system that maximizes community self-reliance and social justice."

PROFESSORS ANNE C. BELLOWS AND M.W. HAMM
Journal of Nutrition Education and Behavior

adding a food-based charity donation to your local food gift this holiday?

Get involved with community gardens (see facing page), a win-win situation that allows low-income neighbors to both connect and feed themselves. Start a community garden yourself on an unused farm, an empty lot, or your neighbor's land. Engage community members, such as immigrants, who may even have an agricultural background, to join.

Support farm-to-school and school garden programs (see page 207) that also provide healthful food to those in need.

Both private- and government-funded local food policy councils are excellent at leveraging public policy resources to improve connections between local food and food security. For more information, contact the Community Food Security Coalition and read Mark Winne's book, *Closing the Food Gap: Resetting the Table in the Land of Plenty.* (See Recommended Reading.)

KEEP BIODIVERSITY ALIVE

In the past 100 years, 93 percent of Native American crop varieties have disappeared from cultivation. Much of this has happened since World War II, when the "green revolution" took root and high-production farming systems became more widespread. (The term "green" is really a misnomer here, since the practices it fostered are based on synthetic chemicals and biotechnology.) Cultivars of plants and breeds of animals were selected for their ability to grow quickly, produce bumper crops, resist disease, and hold up well during transport. The result is a shrinking variety of foods that are not only mediocre and flavorless, but also raised in ways that are detrimental to our environment. All this puts our planet, palate, and food security in jeopardy.

Today a strong movement is afoot to revive a wide variety of cultivars and breeds. You can become a part of it by educating yourself and working to preserve the diversity of plants and animals, many of which are unique to certain regions and have historical significance, as well.

Start with eating-based conservation by simply buying, eating, and savoring unusual cultivars and breeds, especially those traditionally used in your region. Revive our regional foodsheds by preparing local foods using

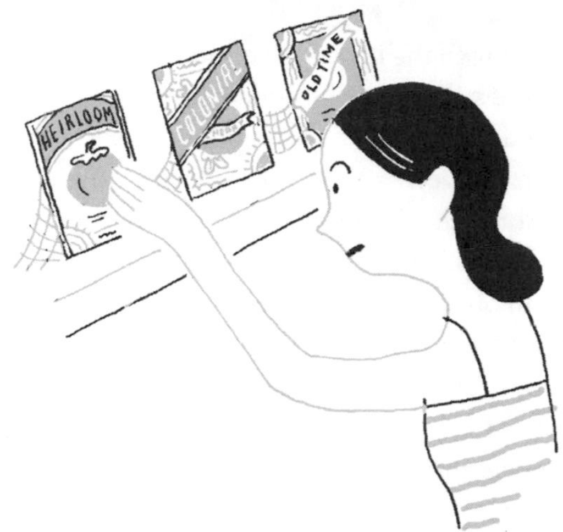

traditional techniques with (or without) your own twist.

Connect with botanical gardens, garden clubs, and conservation groups. Check out Slow Food's RAFT Alliance (see Resources) which initiates and supports conservation, education, promotion, and regional networking projects, or its Ark of Taste, a catalog of over 200 foods in danger of extinction.

Look for heirloom and heritage breeds, then grow or raise your own. Find regional seed catalogs or exchanges, especially those like Seeds of Change and Seed Savers Exchange, that specialize in heirloom varieties (see Resources). Visit the Web site for Heritage Foods USA to find out more about heritage meats, some of which may be raised near you.

Gary Paul Nabhan, Southwest-based author, food and farming advocate, rural lifeways folklorist, and conservationist, is a champion of the work surrounding biodiversity. He also saves the rich stories connected with heritage foods on his Web site (see Resources).

GARDEN OR WORK ON A FARM

Community gardens, popular almost everywhere, are a superb way to connect with local projects or simply learn how to grow your own food. In urban settings, these estimated 10,000 collaborative gardens transform empty lots into green living spaces. Many are too small to be listed on national databases, so ask around your neighborhood or call government offices, garden centers, or community groups. Or start your own (follow the link to the American Community Gardening Association in Resources).

Volunteer to help bring in the harvest at a farm that is requesting volunteers through a local food initiative. Or take it one step further and become a WWOOF volunteer through World Wide Opportunities on Organic Farms. You'll barter a minimum of 25 hours a week for room and board on an organic farm geared toward supporting an educational experience for its volunteers. For more information, visit their Web site (see Resources).

BUILD A FARM-FRIENDLY COMMUNITY

Work to support and foster farming in your region (and our country) by advocating for ecologically sound farms and community-friendly public policies.

Join a local agricultural commission or committee that brings farmers and others together to create an environment in which farm businesses can flourish. Talk with community planners, land trusts, and other community groups to ensure that the needs of local farmers are considered. Make sure your town's zoning bylaws and tax structures are fair to farm businesses. Encourage passage of a "right to farm" policy. Encourage towns to provide free space for farmers' markets. The UNH Cooperative Extension and the New Hampshire Coalition for Sustaining Agriculture have a terrific checklist called "Is Your Town Farm Friendly?" (see Resources).

CHANGING OUR FOOD SYSTEM

Creating a healthier food system — what the food and agriculture writer Michael Pollan calls "sun-driven" rather than cheap oil–driven — is not just a dream. But it requires major policy changes to help cure some of the most pressing crises of our time. Our current food system, supported by once-cheap oil, contributes up to 37 percent of greenhouse gases (by some estimates). Industrial agriculture is second only to cars in use of fossil fuel, and is a major contributor to climate change. Food produced by our current system is also fattening us beyond recognition, clogging our hearts and the health system, degrading local economies and our land, and leaving us with flavorless food. We need to rethink how we produce food and work for policies that advocate those changes. So let's get going!

Find out about public and private funding programs for farmland protection, farm business training, and transitioning to more ecological farming practices. Help create a community land trust that helps make land more affordable for farmers. One example is the exceptional E. F. Schumacher Society that spearheaded a community land trust in my region as well as a groundbreaking local currency. (For information, see the Web link in Resources).

Join existing efforts to advocate for local, state, and federal legislation that support farmers and farming, policies that favor purchase of local farm products by state institutions, and regulatory framework that encourages direct farm-to-consumer sales. Write letters to the editor of your local paper, contact local legislators, and track local food legislation in your state through an online organization. Join and volunteer for organizations that support federal policies — such as the Farm Bill — that have the power to encourage sustainable, localized systems. (See Resources for Web links to the National Sustainable Agriculture Coalition, American Farmland Trust, regional Sustainable Agriculture Working Groups (SAWG), and more.)

TRANSFORM OUR FUTURE THROUGH THE NEXT GENERATION

Support the sustainable chefs and farmers of the future. If the next generation farms sustainably and enjoys and supports local food, then our battle is won. Currently 2 million farmers feed 300 million Americans, and the average farmer is 55 years old. We need to build a country of young, highly skilled, sustainable farmers. Do some research to find culinary and agricultural schools with programs that emphasize sustainable agriculture and local food programs in their curricula. Visit the restaurants of culinary schools that emphasize local foods. (Or attend one and work to change it from the inside.) Chefs have helped push for extraordinary change. Teach the children in your life to appreciate local food and farms. Shop, serve, and savor local food with them. Visit farms. For more information, contact Chefs Collaborative (see Resources).

Engage in a farm-to-school program. A year of visiting school kitchens has shown me firsthand that processed, fatty, and salty foods still dominate our school kitchens. But change is on the way. It's not an easy road, but farm-to-school programs are bringing local, farm-fresh foods into school cafeterias. Support one near you by joining a committee to shape federally mandated

SOMETIMES YOU HAVE TO GET OUT TO THE FARM TO GET THE CONNECTION

A city mom visiting a dairy farm was watching a suckling calf while holding her infant in her arms.

"So that's where we get milk from!" she commented.

"Same as we do," the farmer replied, looking right back at her.

"A-ha," responded the mom, smiling.

Seminal lessons and connections await you on the farm. Some are obvious a-ha moments like that one; others are environmental, culinary, scientific, visceral, and aesthetic. However brief, it's easy to internalize your connection to the farmer, the farm, and its natural surroundings when you visit.

school wellness policy, becoming part of a school board, or supporting beleaguered food-service staff hindered by government policies and lack of proper funding for healthy foods. Most states now have farm-to-school programs connecting local farmers with schools, a win for both.

A book I developed for school food-service staff, *Fresh from the Farm: The Massachusetts Farm to School Cookbook*, is useful and free online. It includes school-tested recipes and educational information on buying and preparing farm-fresh foods, as well as how to connect with local farms. Visit Ann Cooper, the self-described "renegade lunch lady," online and read her book, *Lunch Lessons*. Also visit the Web site of the National Farm to School Network to find resources near you. Its regional agencies and national staff provide free training and technical assistance, information services, networking, and support for policy, media, and marketing activities. For links to these Web sites, see Resources.

Connect with or start a school garden. When kids play a part in growing their own food, they're more likely to eat and enjoy it. Hundreds of schools across the country have created school gardens, some inspired by Alice Waters' project, *The Edible Schoolyard*. Her online resource has information on how to get started. Some companies will even come and set up a school garden or greenhouse for a fee. (Start raising money, PTAs!) Visit Slow Food USA for their Slow Food in Schools and Slow Food on Campus programs.

Growing Healthy Kids

"It doesn't matter where you come from or whether you get As or Ds, everyone has an equal chance for success out on the farm. I've seen youths who struggle with the heat and weeds out on the farm but take on a whole new attitude after they work at the farmers' market. Suddenly, when they're selling food that they grew to their neighbors or taking vegetables home to their families and teaching them how to cook, they gain a sense of what they have accomplished. All those hours of work take on a whole new meaning, and the pride that they feel in the vegetables they are selling and donating is tremendous."

CAMMY WATTS

The Food Project, Director of Education and Advocacy

Bring local food and farm education into the classroom in your school with the numerous resources available, some of which need to be adapted to local food and sustainability issues. Start with work from the Center for Ecoliteracy, a Bay area organization that provides tools, ideas, and support for combining hands-on experience in the natural world with curricular innovation in K–12 education and offers resources and expertise to support the sustainability movement in K–12 schools across the nation. Agriculture in the Classroom provides state contacts and lesson plans for integrating lessons emphasizing the importance of agriculture into the classroom. Your local cooperative extension or 4-H club may have ideas on how to get local kids engaged with farmers. And of course, support efforts to help school classes visit farms near them.

Connect our children with educational projects that take them from the garden (or farm) to market and teach them to become engaged citizens. The Food Project, a nonprofit organization based in and around the Boston area has championed work with young people to build a local agricultural system. They've created and supported replicable models that engage kids in growing food for low-income neighborhood farmers' markets and much more. Project participants work a farm that donates 40 percent of its food to feed those in need; they also work one day a week in a hunger relief agency.

Engage college students in helping to shape the food system. Farm-to-school programs, campus CSAs, and much more are available to college students interested in local, sustainable food. The Real Food Challenge has a multitude of resources and networks on how to get engaged in the local food movement, everything from Campus Food to farm workers' rights and food policy.

Encourage a youth movement. The Slow Food Youth Movement has an international focus on strengthening a network of young farmers, producers, students, chefs, and activists.

See Resources beginning on page 227 for Web links and more information on any of these ideas.

ENGAGE IN ON-FARM EDUCATION

All the lessons of life can be found on a farm, and every region has opportunities to get out to a farm and learn them. Take a casual trip or visit one of the many farms with education components nationwide; some are ad hoc, while others are formal educational programs.

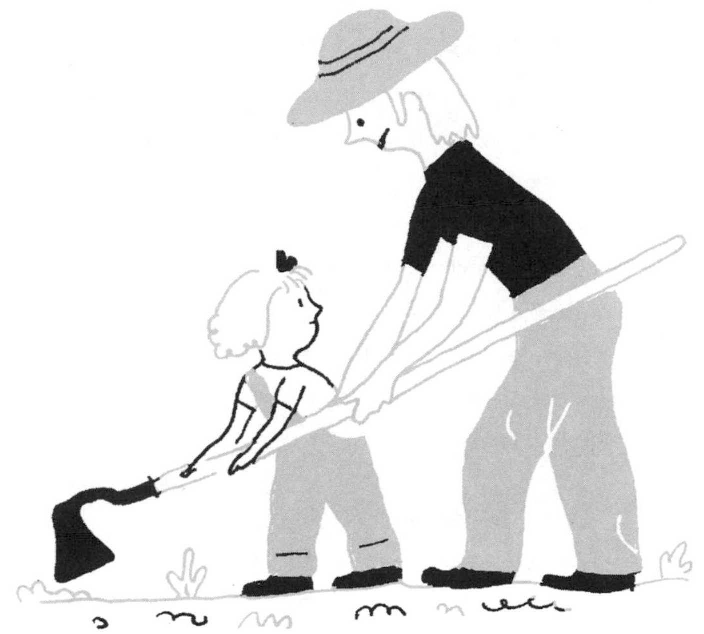

Watch and listen or learn tangible lessons by engaging in farm work, such as planting and harvesting, milking a goat or building a chicken coop, or learning traditional food preservation techniques such as cheese making or putting up jam.

In a broader sense, a good farm visit teaches adults and kids about being part of a closed-loop system — a model of sustainability that considers the whole, rather than just the parts. It connects us to our environment and teaches us about becoming producers, contributors, and recyclers in a culture driven by consumption and waste.

School farm visits are best initiated by garnering the enthusiasm of the teacher and administration before making the farm match. Kids with different learning styles, who may not succeed in a traditional academic environment, may thrive on a farm. Farm education gives them an opportunity to learn the same skills they'll need in the classroom and in their lives. It teaches patience, especially programs that follow plants from seed to harvest through the seasons. Farm visits also show kids that farms aren't about nostalgia but are working businesses. Well-done on-site farm education does a service to farms by emphasizing the importance of agriculture. (It may also provide an additional revenue stream for farmers struggling to survive.)

Singing to the Trees

In mid-May, when the apple trees are in full flower, I attend Breezy Hill Orchard's annual all-stops-out farm party. There's a long buffet with fresh food galore, including plenty of cider for 200 to 400 guests, who arrive at the farm to dance and wassail the trees, an old Celtic tradition. Then, bearing candles, with a 15-piece Balkan brass band leading the way, we walk in a long procession to an old apple tree, with branches wide enough to form a small room. With lyrics provided, we wassail the tree, then place our candles in its branches, along with last year's cider, some dipped in bread, some soaking the ground to ensure next year's harvest.

Education departments in each state have their own criteria for fitting gardening and farming into all aspects of the school curriculum. In the summer, consider farm-based camps or burgeoning farm- and garden-education programs at traditional camps.

A growing database of programs and sites, as well as lessons, activities, and materials, is available online at the Farm-Based Education Association (see Resources).

A secret about sustainable community advocacy is that giving is about getting back, too. So if your work feeds you in some way, you're on the right path.

START OR SUPPORT A FARMERS' MARKET, CSA, OR BUYING CLUB

Your local farmers' market may need volunteers on market day to help market managers and farmers, or for longer term work, such as serving on the market board or committee. Or, they may need your skills. A graphic designer can help with a sign, ad, or logo. A writer might help a market clearly define their rules, edit a newsletter, or write press releases.

If there isn't a market near you, get one going, but don't take the process lightly. Start by engaging not just farmers but also surrounding businesses and community members, in addition to your state farmers' market association. For more information, visit the Web site of the Farmers' Market Coalition (see Resources).

Robyn Van En spearheaded the CSA movement in America with a small, handwritten book still published by the Robyn Van En Center at Wilson College. The center traces and supports CSAs and can steer you in the right direction (see Resources).

While visiting or vacationing far from home, be sure to seek out regional local food specialties, such as wine, wild rice, and cranberries, to savor or to take home.

SEEK OUT OR START LOCAL FOOD-BASED EVENTS

In the mid 1990s, a band of local food folks and I ran a series of moveable feasts throughout my county in western Massachusetts. These were simple, inexpensive meals meant to celebrate the local harvest. They introduced dialog about local food and even spurred the formation of a butternut squash cooperative.

There are many seasonal food events around the country. Although some may have drifted away from the local food emphasis — by say, introducing feedlot pork into pig roasts or Florida corn into a Fourth of July local food party — they can be easily redirected to bring in local food themes. Whether you are volunteering to raise money for your school or holding a wine tasting, be sure to invite and engage farmers by paying them a fair price for their food. Or create your own event at home or out in the community. Track local food events through Local Harvest, connect with the 100-mile-diet groups emerging across the country, or join a Slow Food RAFT Picnic (see Resources).

BECOME AN AGRITOURIST

When you visit friends and family or go on vacation, travel like a locavore. You'll find out where to eat the best food, you'll meet the nicest people, and you'll have a savory trip, too.

Get a picture of the region by visiting farms and farmers' markets instead of (or along with) sites and

VISIT A FARM AND CHANGE YOUR WORLDVIEW

Locavores of all stripes will tell you the seeds of their local food activism took root on a farm. Visiting a farm — whether it's to pick berries, take a class in cheese making, or look at a historical herb garden — can be transformative.

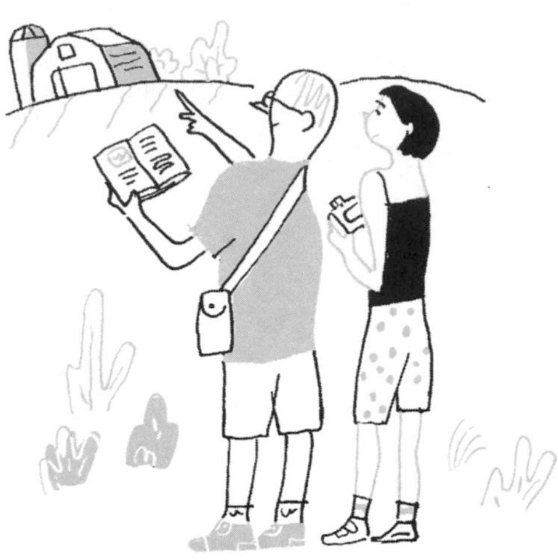

monuments. We often associate this kind of agritourism with distant lands, but plenty of places in the United States can offer a taste of distinctive local foods. Seek out agricultural fairs, farmers' markets, farm-centered education centers, and whatever wonderful quirks a region has to offer.

START SOMEWHERE

You don't have to be a gonzo local activist to jump in here. There aren't any food police to monitor your political correctness; the level of the engagement is your call. Whatever works for you works.

So get a handle on the framework for the local food movement using this book and its resources, ask around or check out any of the connections listed in the Resources section, work solo, get connected with an existing organization, or provide leadership for a small initiative, growing it in a manner that sustains its participants, effectiveness, and financial support.

You're most effective if your approach resonates with you personally: this will help you to forge ahead. It may help to go where your skills and interests lie. Entrepreneurs interested in the local economy might work with their chamber of commerce or economic development agency, tree huggers with land trusts, foodies through feasts. Or use your community work to balance your work life, like an accountant tired of deskwork who gets her hands in the soil on weekends.

Start with your own local food journey, savoring it with friends and family, taking it out into your community, your region, and the world — eating your way to a better and more delicious planet.

Appendix

KEY EVENTS IN LOCAL FOOD HISTORY

Are you a locavore? Or an activist opening one of the windows to community engagement in the previous chapter? Whatever our engagement, we're all part of something bigger than ourselves: the local food movement. And it's easier to get and stay involved if we have a little context. Of course, there's no perfect chronological order for the events that make up the history of this contemporary movement, because many of them converged, overlapping throughout a short time period. So don't take what's here too literally. Rather, consider it more of a crash course. While I've tended to cite more national groups here, local and regional groups too numerous to name here have led the way.

Rodale spurs interest in small-scale sustainable farming.

Wendell Berry and other environmentalists focus on the importance of eating as "an agricultural act."

Back-to-the-land movement focuses on homesteading and self-sufficiency.

Alice Waters' Chez Panisse opens in Berkeley, California, emphasizing fresh, regional foods.

In *Diet for a Small Planet,* Frances Moore Lappé awakens us to how every food choice helps to create the world we want.

Americans become obsessed with new foods and food combinations, expanding their diet.

World travel, international cookbooks, and immigrant populations broaden American tastes.

A growing interest in healthy eating and whole food procurement takes hold. Bulk-buying health food clubs emerge, some of which will become community food co-ops that will later focus on local foods. The concept plants the seed for local food-buying clubs later on.

Health research continues to support consumption of more produce, which is emphasized more in shopping venues. Vegetarianism flourishes.

CSAs (community supported agriculture farms) take root in the United States and boom, starting with Indian Line Farm in Massachusetts — all putting a face on farming by bringing farmer and consumer together.

Numerous farmers' markets are born and boom, too, greatly influencing restaurants, chefs, and home cooks, as well as invigorating neighborhoods.

Grassroots food and small farms advocacy groups spring up, initiated by environmentalists, foodies, and farmers.

Local food is linked to healthy living local economies, some inspired by E.F. Schumacher Society and Judy Wicks at the White Dog Restaurant in Philadelphia, Pennsylvania.

Farmers and entrepreneurs create more quality, value-added farm products, such as artisanal cheeses.

Farmers bring to market more heirloom produce and heritage breeds, expanding food diversity and pushing back against monoculture.

Growing and saving seeds from heirloom varieties becomes popular among gardeners.

Smaller farms emerge as farming becomes radically consolidated, some assisted by nonprofits and federal programs, like SARE, as well as agricultural extension and state agricultural programs.

Sustainable agriculture and Buy Local campaigns emerge nationwide, many jump-started by FoodRoutes programs, which provide models for regional initiatives.

Demand for organic food skyrockets and big corporations jump on board.

Restaurant chefs focus more on farm-based food and introducing the public to local foods, with Chefs Collaborative leading the way.

Distress about the culinary industrial complex, as emphasized in books like *Fast Food Nation* and *The Omnivore's Dilemma*, raise health concerns and engage interest in sustainable agriculture.

Food security and fresh local food are linked in projects nationwide. The Food Security Coalition is born, as is the farm-to-school movement, supported by the National Farm to School Network.

A dazzling array of sustainable foods appears on the market with words like *grass-fed* and, well, *sustainable* everything, often loosely labeled.

Community vegetable gardens multiply, bringing better food into rural neighborhoods while engaging and invigorating communities.

Slow Food International jumps the ocean and settles in the United States, inspiring Americans' intense interest in local food and reviving biodiversity.

Foundations like Kellogg, regional grassroots conferences, and forums like the Baum Forum focus on creating a closer farm-to-table connection.

Land trusts take an interest in agricultural land preservation as part of a healthy diverse landscape.

A barrage of seasonal and farmers' market cookbooks hit the marketplace.

The new global economy, organic standards, and the farm bills inspire activists to galvanize, reexamine, and push against food raised without concern for people, animals, or the planet.

School garden programs teach students about fresh, local food, many inspired by Alice Waters' Edible Schoolyard.

Local food goes mainstream and words like *local, native,* and *heirloom* pop up everywhere, sometimes without much consideration to fact.

Marian Nestle's links to healthy and local food and her book, *Food Politics*, shows us how unhealthful choices are made for us and forces us to look at how *bounty* does not mean *health.*

The rise of GMOs and corporate-owned terminator seeds, banned in many parts of the word, raise concerns.

Vandana Shiva's *Stolen Harvest: The Hijacking of the Global Food Supply* teaches us that the global food system is not about good food for everyone.

Books like *The Hundred Mile Diet* and *Animal, Vegetable, Miracle* personalize local food and help mainstream the local food movement.

Baby boomers' children become interested in local food, work on sustainable farms in projects like WWOOF, and push for better school food on campus.

RAFT (Renewing America's Food Traditions), a collaboration reviving locally adapted seeds, is born. Gary Nabhan writes eloquently about biodiversity.

Writer Michael Pollan, poet laureate of the local food movement, publishes a *New York Times* magazine article, "Farmer in Chief," outlining for the new president the creation of a sustainable regional food system.

On-farm educational programs inspire children and adults to reexamine where their food comes from.

The economy tightens and Americans become more interested in gardening, cooking at home, and economic ways to eat well.

Numerous Web sites and Listservs are born, steering Americans to local food information.

First Lady Michelle Obama plants a White House vegetable garden, sparking interest in gardening and healthful local foods.

LOCAL FOOD AND SUSTAINABILITY GLOSSARY

Plenty of words like *organic* and *naturally grown* are bandied about without regard to their actual meaning. Understanding their definitions and their local food context will help you to make choices that are right for you.

Agribusiness The term literally means agriculture and business, hardly a negative combination, because farms are businesses. But for those interested in local foods and a healthy environment, it has a negative connotation. The word is generally used to describe large-scale industrial corporate farms, major polluters and energy consumers, often producing low-quality "cheap" food at great expense to us all.

Agritourism Tourism with an agricultural bent, such as visiting farmers' markets, pick-your-own farms, and wineries.

Artisanal Food made by hand or in a traditional way, often in small batches.

Biodiversity The variation of life forms within a given ecosystem, often used to measure its health.

Biodynamic farming Organic *plus*. Initiated by Rudolf Steiner, about 20 years before the development of organic farming, nonchemical biodynamic farming uses a variety of integrated holistic methods, many of which cross over with organic farming but also utilize the forces of nature, such as the cycles of the moon.

Bovine growth hormone Hormone injected into diary cows to increase milk production, called recombinant bovine somatotropin (rBST). Because of evidence that it may have harmful effects, it's banned in all countries but the United States, South Africa, and Mexico. The hormone shortens a cow's lifespan and makes it more susceptible to disease.

Buying club (or single-ingredient CSA) See page 68.

CAFO See Feedlot.

Carbon footprint How much greenhouse gas it takes to produce a specific item or sustain your lifestyle. It's hard to measure, but local food has a smaller footprint than food traveling through the conventional food system. (See Food miles.)

Certified humane Produced according to guidelines that are concerned with the welfare of animals.

Certified naturally grown An eco-label with guidelines, including farm inspections and random residue testing, for farmers who grow using organic methods but have chosen not to become USDA certified organic.

CSA (Community Supported Agriculture) See page 48.

Diversified farm A farm that does more than one thing. Smaller sustainable farms often tend toward diversity, whereas larger agribusiness farms do not. (The opposite of a monoculture farm; see page 224.)

Eco-label A label for products that cause less damage to the environment. Some are enforced and verified by third party agencies, others are self-awarded. For more information visit the Web site for the Consumers Union Guide to Environmental Labels (see Resources).

Endangered foods Endangered foods are ingredients that may become extinct, as many of our foods already have. (The Slow Food Ark of Taste is working to preserve them. See Resources.)

Factory farm Large-scale industrial farm, such as a giant feedlot farm (see Feedlot). These farms are major polluters and energy hogs.

Farm Bill Federal legislation, renewed about every five years. The Food, Conservation, and Energy Act, last enacted in 2008, governs most agriculture and related programs. Local food activists advocate for a rehauled farm bill that refocuses on regionalized food systems, supports sustainable farms, and provides funding for better access to fresh food for all, instead of subsidizing the existing industrial food complex.

Farmers' market See page 23.

Feedlot The confined animal feeding operation (CAFO), also called a feedlot, is a method used on industrial farms to raise as many animals as possible in a small space (we're talking *thousands* of animals), for maximum profit. Animals are generally fed food that is unnatural to their diet and are kept in confined spaces rather than open pastures.

Food co-op Member-owned food stores that grew out of the desire to buy whole foods in bulk at a reduced price. These are now often stores with a "natural foods" bent, many of which make a strong commitment to local food procurement.

Foodie Anyone seriously interested in food.

Food miles How many miles it takes from farm to point of purchase. It is one way to assess the environmental impact of food. Our food takes an average of 1,500 miles to reach us, 27 times higher than food from local sources. In short: local food uses fewer food miles.

Foodshed Your foodshed encompasses the area your food comes from — farm to table. The conventional contemporary foodshed is global. The local food movement strives for regional foodsheds, sometimes within 100 miles of where you live, often more.

Food system Everything from farm to table, including food production, processing, distribution, consumption and waste management. (See Sustainable community food system.)

Food traditions Cultural, regional, and familial food traditions preserve an essential part of our civilization. Gardening, buying local foods, preparing heirloom regional and family dishes, and celebrating annual harvest celebrations are ways to do so.

Free-range The term usually refers to poultry and the eggs they produce, and means the birds have *access* to the outdoors, but aren't necessarily wandering freely on the farm. The USDA considers five minutes a day adequate.

Genetically modified food (GMO) An animal or plant that has been genetically engineered. They are banned in many parts of the world, such as Europe and Japan, because the jury is still out on their safety, but they are legal here. Labeling them would at least give consumers a chance to make their own choices. Non-GMO foods are not genetically engineered.

Geographical indication Sometimes abbreviated to GI, this is a name or sign used on certain products that come from a specific geographical location or origin (e.g., a town, region, or country). The use of a GI may act as a certification that the product possesses certain qualities, or enjoys a certain reputation, because of its geographical origin.

Grass-fed or -pastured Raised on pasture. For more specifics, see Meat and Poultry on page 170.

Heirloom vegetables and fruits Refers to open-pollinated produce more commonly grown during earlier times, generally 50 years or more ago, and not commonly used in contemporary agriculture. (See page 192.) Modern varieties are bred for their durability (ability to pack and ship well), not necessarily their flavor. By contrast, heirlooms may sometimes look irregular, but often taste great. In many places, the popularly of heirloom vegetables has brought back biodiversity in the marketplace.

Heritage breeds Rare or endangered breeds of livestock, raised for their flavor, their cultural significance, and to preserve genetic diversity.

Holistic management A holistic decision-making framework with a monitoring system for farmers to establish and meet their farm's long-term financial and biological farm goals.

Integrated pest management (IPM) Often a bridge from conventional to organic agriculture, this system combines a variety of pest control methods, such as pest predators and natural deterrents, in order to limit the use of chemical pesticides.

Local and regional Many locavores define *local* as within 100–150 miles. In this book, local means that it is from your immediate area. I don't define it by mileage, as growing regions don't work as the fly crows, but rather by the lay of the land. Agricultural regions are sometimes called foodsheds. The supposition in this book is that it is good to buy your food as close to home as possible.

Local food Food grown within your foodshed, see Foodshed.

Local food movement Movement to support an alternative food system that is locally based, delicious, ecologically responsible, and self-reliant. This broad movement covers food production, processing, distribution, and consumption, often embracing regional foods and food traditions, all integrated to enrich the environmental, economic, and social health of a particular place.

Local food systems An alternative food system, based locally and regionally, rather than globally. A local food system puts "a face on farming" by developing relationships along the food chain, from farm to fork. It tends to support smaller, more environmentally and community-friendly farms, which also keep their hard-earned dollars close to home rather than in a few corporate hands. See food system.

Locavore You or anyone who seeks out and savors locally grown and raised foods. Coined in San Francisco in 2005, *locavore* was the word of the year in the 2007 New Oxford American Dictionary.

Monoculture The replacement of a diverse ecosystem with a single species or crop. This kind of farming depletes the land and makes crops more susceptible to disease, requiring more chemical intervention — think fields of a single potato cultivar as far as the eye can see, growing in soil that doesn't look or feel much like soil at all. (For the opposite, see Diversified farm.)

Native plants Plants grown in your area prior to European settlement.

Natural Essentially a meaningless word. According to the USDA it means meat and poultry products can only undergo minimal processing and cannot contain what they consider artificial ingredients, such as colors or flavors. It doesn't mean they are raised in a sustainable manner, *or that they are free of hormones and antibiotics.*

Nose to tail Term used to mean the entire animal was used in cooking, not just the prime cuts. It's a more ecological way of cooking used by chefs interested in sustainable foods.

Organic Since 1995, to be called organic, a farm must meet USDA organic standards and certification criteria. The National Organic Standards Board states, "Organic agriculture is an ecological production management system that promotes and enhances biodiversity, biological cycles and soil biological activity. It is based on minimal use of off-farm inputs and on management practices that restore, maintain and enhance ecological harmony." This means: no synthetic fertilizers, chemicals, sewage sludge, GMOs, or irradiation. Animals cannot be treated with hormones or antibiotics, must have access to pasture, and be fed organically grown feed with no animal byproducts. Since this has become a government certification there has been major pushback from large corporate farming interests to loosen standards. *Note that many farms use organic methods but are not certified.* See also Local vs. Organic on page 13.

Organic farms Farms using organic methods. Organic farms can be small or large agribusiness corporate farms. (See certified naturally grown; Local vs. Organic on page 13.)

BEYOND ORGANIC

After 1995, when the government developed organic standards, many farms that had been growing organically or using even stricter standards decided not to become certified, for a variety of reasons, including the massive amounts of paperwork involved and fact that the term organic was being co-opted by big business. Those that go beyond the USDA certification but are not certified are sometimes called "Beyond Organic."

Pasteurization A process to kill bacteria by heating milk to 145°F for half an hour or 161°F for 15 seconds. For ultra-pasturization, milk is heated to 285°F for 1 to 2 seconds.

Pasture raised See What's the Story with Grass? on page 171.

Real food Whole unprocessed food that is produced sustainably.

Seasonal In season in a specific region. Seasonal shopping and cooking is vital to a locavore's life and eating pleasure.

Slow food An international organization and grassroots movement that encourages a more mindful way of eating and living. It's about sharing and savoring food that is sustainably produced with respect for people, the planet, and our communities. See Slow Food USA in Resources.

Sustainable community food system What we are striving for! A collaborative network that encompasses all the components it takes to bring food from farm to table. A sustainable community food system integrates all of these — farming, food processing, distribution, and consumption as well as waste management — in order to create a better food supply. The result is better social, environmental, and economic health for the community.

A sustainable community food system includes a base of sustainable farms with good working conditions for farm labor, direct links between farmers and consumers, better access to fresh food for all, healthy food and agriculture businesses, as well as policies that support all this.

Sustainable farming or agricultural practices Ideally sustainable farms provide a secure living for farmers, while supporting a healthy environment, community, and just treatment for all. Many different agricultural techniques can be used to help make food production sustainable, enriching rather than destroying our natural resources. There is also a cultural and social implication that those who grow our food sustainably maintain and nourish a good working environment, practice fair labor practices and humane treatment of animals, and produce food that is healthy and sustains life itself. The modern sustainable agriculture movement grew out of a reaction to high-chemical, high-crop yield industrial farming, which escalated rapidly in the late 20th century.

Sustainable foods Foods produced using renewable resources. Sustainably raised foods maintain and even replenish people, animals, our economy and, of course, our environment.

Terroir Often associated with wine and cheese. In the local food world, it has come to mean "a taste of place." Food grown in a specific region may have its own distinctive character.

Traceability Ability to trace your food to where it originated.

Value-added foods Farm foods that have value added to them through any kind of process, such as ice cream produced from milk or butternut squash that has been peeled. Value-added products sell for more than their straight-from-the-farm equivalents.

Virtuous globalization Slow Food calls it "virtuous globalization" when the power of a global market can be used to defend an endangered local food or food culture.

Working landscape Our farms.

RESOURCES

100 Mile Diet
www.100milediet.org

Agriculture in the Classroom
United States Department of Agriculture
202-720-2727
www.agclassroom.org

Alternative Farming Systems Information Center
United States Department of Agriculture
301-504-6559
http://afsic.nal.usda.gov

American Community Gardening Association
877-275-2242
http://communitygarden.org

American Farmland Trust
202-331-7300
www.farmland.org

American Grassfed Association
877-774-7277
www.americangrassfed.org

American Pastured Poultry Producers Association
888-662-7772
www.apppa.org

Amy Cotler
413-232-7174
www.amycotler.com
Download *Fresh From the Farm: The Massachusetts Farm to School Cookbook*

Ann Cooper
www.chefann.com
The "Renegade Lunch Lady"

ATTRA — National Sustainable Agriculture Information Service
800-346-9140
http://attra.ncat.org

Baum Forum
718-884-5716
www.baumforum.org

Berkshire Grown
413-528-0041
http://berkshiregrown.org

Billie Best
www.billiebest.com
10 essays on the politics of farming

Biodynamic Farming and Gardening Association
888-516-7797
www.biodynamics.com

Blue Ocean Institute
516-922-9500
www.blueoceaninstitute.com

A Campaign for Real Milk
The Weston A. Price Foundation
202-363-4394
www.realmilk.com

Center for Ecoliteracy
510-845-4595
www.ecoliteracy.org

Center for Food and Justice
Urban & Environmental Policy Institute, Occidental College
323-341-5099
http://departments.oxy.edu/uepi/cfj

Center for Urban Education about Sustainable Agriculture
415-291-3276
www.cuesa.org

Chefs Collaborative
617-236-5200
www.chefscollaborative.org

Chowhound
www.chowhound.com

Community Alliance with Family Farmers
530-756-8518
http://caff.org

Community Food Security Coalition
503-954-2970
http://foodsecurity.org

Community Involved In Sustaining Agriculture (CISA)
866-965-7100
www.buylocalfood.com
Provides an information bulletin entitled "Community Supported Agriculture for the Workplace: A Guide for Developing Workplace Community Supported Agriculture Distributions"

ContainerGardeningTips.com
www.containergardeningtips.com

Cooperative Extension System
www.csrees.usda.gov/Extension

Culinate
877-873-9306
www.culinate.com

Dowd's Guide to American Wine Trails
http://americanwinetrails.blogspot.com

The E. F. Schumacher Society
413-528-1737
www.smallisbeautiful.org

Earth Pledge
212-725-6611
www.earthpledge.org

Eat Local Challenge
http://eatlocalchallenge.com

Eat Well Guide
212-991-1858
www.eatwellguide.org

Economic Research Service
United States Department of Agriculture
202-694-5050
www.ers.usda.gov

Edible Communities Publications
800-652-4217
www.ediblecommunities.com
Regional local food magazines

Edible Landscaping
434-361-9134
www.ediblelandscaping.com

The Edible Schoolyard
Chez Panisse Foundation and Martin Luther King Jr. Middle School
510-558-1335
www.edibleschoolyard.org

Environmental Commons
info@environmentalcommons.org
http://environmentalcommons.org

The Ethicurean
www.ethicurean.com
Good information on the web about starting a meat CSA; has full descriptions, although the circumstances vary from place to place.

FactoryFarm.org
Food & Water Watch
www.factoryfarm.org

Farm Locator
Rodale Institute
610-683-1400
www.rodaleinstitute.org/farm_locator

Farm to College
FoodRoutes Network
570-673-3398
www.foodroutes.org/farmtocollege.jsp

Farm to School
Center for Food & Justice, Urban & Environmental Policy Institute
323-341-5095
www.farmtoschool.org

Farm to Table
505-473-1004
www.farmtotablenm.org

Farm-Based Education Association
www.farmbasededucation.org

Farmers' Market Coalition
www.farmersmarketcoalition.org

FarmPolicy.com
217-356-2269
www.farmpolicy.com

FarmtoCollege.org
Community Food Security Coalition
570-658-2265
http://farmtocollege.org

Farmworker Justice
202-293-5420
www.fwjustice.org

Food Alliance
503-493-1066
www.foodalliance.org

Food Family Farming Foundation (Chef Ann Cooper: The Renegade Lunch Lady)
631-697-0844
www.foodfamilyfarming.org

Food, Farming, & Community
The Voices Project, Michigan State University Museum
517-432-3358
www.foodfarmingandcommunity.org

The Food Project
info@thefoodproject.org
www.thefoodproject.org

FoodRoutes Network
570-673-3398
www.foodroutes.org

FoodShare Toronto
416-363-6441
www.foodshare.net

Gary Nabhan
www.garynabhan.com

GRACE
212-726-9161
www.gracelinks.org

Greener Choices Eco-Labels Center
Consumer Reports
www.greenerchoices.org/eco-labels

Hartford Food System
860-296-9325
http://hartfordfood.org

Heifer Project International
800-422-0474
www.heifer.org

Heritage Foods USA
212-980-6603
www.heritagefoodsusa.com

Home Food Preservation
Food Safety Program
Pennsylvania State University
http://foodsafety.psu.edu/canningguide.html
Provides the most up-to-date version of the *USDA's Complete Guide to Home Canning and Preserving.*

Institute for Agriculture and Trade Policy
612-870-0453
www.iatp.org

Institute for Responsible Technology
641-209-1765
www.responsibletechnology.org

Just Food
www.justfood.org
Just Food is a nonprofit organization that works to develop a just and sustainable food system in the New York City region.

Leopold Center for Sustainable Agriculture
Iowa State University
515-294-3711
www.leopold.iastate.edu

LocalHarvest
831-475-8150
www.localharvest.org

Michael Pollan
http://michaelpollan.com
Web site of Michael Pollan, author of *In Defense of Food* and *The Omnivore's Dilemma.*

Michigan Food and Farming Systems
517-432-0712
www.miffs.org

Midwest Organic and Sustainable Education Service
715-778-5775
www.mosesorganic.org

National Association of State Departments of Agriculture
202-296-9680
www.nasda.org

National Black Farmers Association
804-691-8528
www.blackfarmers.org

National Center for Home Food Preservation
University of Georgia
www.uga.edu/nchfp

National Cooperative Grocers Association
319-466-9029
www.ncga.coop

National Organic Coalition
www.nationalorganiccoalition.org

National Sustainable Agriculture Coalition
202-547-5754
http://sustainableagriculture.org

Native Seeds/SEARCH
520-622-5561
www.nativeseeds.org

Nebraska Sustainable Agriculture Society
402-525-7794
www.nebsusag.org

New Entry Sustainable Farming Project
Friedman School of Nutrition, Tufts University
978-654-6745
http://nesfp.nutrition.tufts.edu

New York Times Local Food Navigator
http://topics.nytimes.com/top/reference/timestopics/subjects/l/local_food

Northeast Organic Farming Association
203-888-5146
www.nofa.org

Northeast Sustainable Agriculture Working Group
413-323-9878
www.nesawg.org

Nuestras Raíces
413-535-1789
www.nuestras-raices.org

NY Beginning Farmer Project
Cornell University Cooperative Extension
www.nybeginningfarmers.org

Ohio Ecological Food & Farm Association
614-421-2022
www.oeffa.org

Organic Consumers Association
218-226-4164
http://organicconsumers.org

Pennsylvania Association for Sustainable Agriculture
814-349-9856
www.pasafarming.org

People's Grocery
510-652-7607
http://peoplesgrocery.org

PickYourOwn.org
www.pickyourown.org
Find a pick-your-own farm near you.

Real Food Challenge
617-442-1322
http://realfoodchallenge.org

Robyn Van En Center at Wilson College
www.wilson.edu/csasearch/search.asp
National resource center for community supported

agriculture. Includes a searchable database of CSA farms throughout the United States.

The Rural Advancement Foundation International — USA
919-542-1396
www.rafiusa.org

The Rural Coalition
202-628-7160
www.ruralco.org

SAWG (Sustainable Agriculture Working Groups)
See regional listings:
Northeast SAWG
www.nesawg.org
Southern SAWG
www.ssawg.org
Western SAWG
www.westernsawg.org
Midwest SAWG
www.msawg.org

Seafood Watch
Monterey Bay Aquarium
877-229-9990
www.montereybayaquarium.org/cr/seafoodwatch.aspx
Provides a consumer's guide to sustainable seafood.

Seed Savers Exchange
563-382-5990
www.seedsavers.org

Seed Savers Network
www.seedsavers.net

Seeds of Change
888-762-7333
www.seedsofchange.com

Shopper's Guide to Pesticides
Foodnews, Environmental Working Group
www.foodnews.org

Slow Food USA
877-756-8366
http://slowfoodusa.org
Home of Renewing America's Food Traditions, U.S. Ark of Taste, and U.S. Presidia.

Small Planet Institute
617-441-6300
www.smallplanet.org
The online home of Frances Moore Lappé and Anna Lappé.

Small Plot Intensive Farming
http://spinfarming.com

Southern Sustainable Agriculture Working Group
info@ssawg.org
www.ssawg.org

State & Local Food Policy Councils
Drake University
515-271-4956
www.statefoodpolicy.org

Sustainable Agriculture Education Association
saea.contact@gmail.com
http://sustainableaged.org

Sustainable Agriculture Research and Education
www.sare.org

Sustainable Food Center
512-236-0074
www.sustainablefoodcenter.org

Sustainable New Mexico
viva@sustainablenewmexico.org
www.sustainablenewmexico.org

Sustainable Table
212-991-1930
www.sustainabletable.org

United Farm Workers
661-823-6250
http://ufw.org

The United States National Arboretum
www.usna.usda.gov
USDA Plant Hardiness Zone Map

University of New Hampshire Cooperative Extension
http://cecf1.unh.edu/sustainable/farmfrnd.cfm
"Is Your Town Farm Friendly?" checklist

Vermont Fresh Network
802-434-2000
www.vermontfresh.net

Western Sustainable Agriculture Working Group
775-964-1022
www.westernsawg.org

What to Eat
www.whattoeatbook.com
Marion Nestle's blog.

Wholesale and Farmers' Markets
Agricultural Marketing Service
www.ams.usda.gov/farmersmarkets

Wild Food!
wildman@wildmanstevebrill.com
www.wildmanstevebrill.com
Web site of forager "Wildman" Steve Brill.

Wilson College
www.wilson.edu/csasearch
Locate a CSA near you.

Women, Infants, and Children
Food & Nutrition Service
www.fns.usda.gov/wic
Home of the WIC Farmers' Market Nutrition Program

World Wide Opportunities on Organic Farms
www.wwoof.org

Your Backyard Farmer
farmers@yourbackyardfarmer.com
www.yourbackyardfarmer.com

RECOMMENDED READING

Bartholomew, Mel. *Square Foot Gardening: A New Way to Garden in Less Space with Less Work*. Emmaus, PA: Rodale, 2005.

Brownell, Kelly D. and Katherine Battle Horgen. *Food Fight: The Inside Story of the Food Industry, America's Obesity Crisis, & What We Can Do About It.* New York: McGraw Hill, 2004.

Bubel, Mike and Nancy Bubel. *Root Cellaring: Natural Cold Storage of Fruits & Vegetables*. North Adams, MA: Storey, 1991.

Carroll, Ricki. *Home Cheesemaking.* North Adams, MA: Storey, 2002.

Chadwick, Janet. *The Beginner's Guide to Preserving Food at Home*, 3rd ed. North Adams, MA: Storey, 2009.

Chesman, Andrea. *Pickles & Relishes*. North Adams, MA: Storey, 2002.

Chioffi, Nancy and Gretchen Mead. *Keeping the Harvest*. North Adams, MA: Storey, 2002.

Coleman, Eliot. *Four-Season Harvest: Organic Vegetables from Your Home Garden All Year Long*, rev. ed. White River Junction, VT: Chelsea Green, 1999.

———. *The New Organic Grower: A Master's Manual of Tools and Techniques for the Home and Market Gardener*. White River Junction, VT: Chelsea Green, 1995.

Cook, Christopher D. *Diet for a Dead Planet: How the Food Industry is Killing Us*. New York: New Press, 2004.

Cooper, Ann and Lisa M. Holmes. *Lunch Lessons: Changing the Way We Feed Our Children*. New York: Harper Collins, 2006.

Denckla, Tanya L. K. *The Gardener's A–Z Guide to Growing Organic Food*. North Adams, MA: Storey, 2003.

Fallon, Sally and Mary G. Enig. *Nourishing Traditions: The Cookbook that Challenges Politically Correct Nutrition and the Diet Dictocrats*, 2nd ed. Washington, D.C.: New Trends, 2001.

Fromartz, Samuel. *Organic, Inc.: Natural Foods and How They Grew*. Orlando: Hartcourt, 2006.

Gardeners and Farmers of Terre Vivante, The. *Preserving Food without Freezing or Canning: Traditional Techniques Using Salt, Oil, Sugar, Alcohol, Vinegar, Drying, Cold Storage and Lactic Fermentation*. White River Junction, VT: Chelsea Green, 2007.

Gibbons, Euell. *Stalking the Wild Asparagus*. Chambersburg, PA: Alan C. Hood, 1962.

Greene, Janet, Ruth Hertzberg, and Beatrice Vaughan. *Putting Food By*, 4th ed. New York: Plume, 1991.

Grescoe, Taras. *Bottomfeeder: How to Eat Ethically in a World of Vanishing Seafood*. New York: Bloomsbury, 2008.

Gussow, Joan Dye. *This Organic Life: Confessions of a Suburban Homesteader*. White River Junction, VT: Chelsea Green, 2001.

Halweil, Brian. *Eat Here: Reclaiming Homegrown Pleasures in a Global Marketplace*. New York: W. W. Norton, 2004.

Harrison, Kathy. *Just In Case, How to Be Self-Sufficient When the Unexpected Happens*. North Adams, MA: Storey, 2008.

Henderson, Elizabeth and Robyn Van En. *Sharing the Harvest: A Citizen's Guide to Community Support Agriculture*, rev. ed. White River Junction, VT: Chelsea Green, 2007.

Katz, Sandor Ellix. *Wild Fermentation: The Flavor, Nutrition, and Craft of Live-Culture Foods.* White River Junction, VT: Chelsea Green, 2003.

Kingry, Judi and Lauren Devine, eds. *Complete Book of Home Preserving.* Toronto: Robert Rose, 2006.

Kingsolver, Barbara. *Animal, Vegetable, Miracle: A Year of Food Life.* New York: HarperCollins, 2007.

Lappé, Anna and Bryant Terry. *Grub: Ideas for an Urban Organic Kitchen.* New York: Tarcher, 2006.

Lappé, Frances Moore and Anna Lappé. *Hope's Edge: The Next Diet for a Small Planet.* New York: Tarcher, 2002.

Lowenfels, Jeff and Wayne Lewis. *Teaming with Microbes: A Gardener's Guide to the Soil Food Web.* Portland, OR: Timber, 2006.

Madison, Deborah. *Local Flavors: Cooking and Eating from America's Farmers' Markets.* New York: Broadway, 2002.

McClure, Susan. *The Herb Gardener: A Guide for All Seasons.* North Adams, MA: Storey, 1996.

Moreland, Rachel Miller. *Simply in Season: Leader's Study Guide.*
Available from World Community Cookbooks. Visit their website at:
www.worldcommunitycookbook.org

Nabhan, Gary Paul. *Coming Home to Eat: The Pleasures and Politics of Local Foods.* New York: Norton, 2002.

———, ed. *Renewing America's Food Traditions: Saving and Savoring the Continent's Most Endangered Foods.* White River Junction, VT: Chelsea Green, 2008

Nestle, Marion. *Food Politics: How the Food Industry Influences Nutrition and Health.* Berkeley: University of California, 2002.

Ogden, Shepherd. *Step by Step Organic Vegetable Gardening.* New York: Harper Collins, 1992.

Parsons, Russ. *How to Pick a Peach: The Search for Flavor from Farm to Table.* Boston: Houghton Mifflin, 2007.

Pears, Pauline. *Rodale's Illustrated Encyclopedia of Organic Gardening.* New York: DK, 2002.

Planck, Nina. *Real Food: What to Eat and Why.* New York: Bloomsbury, 2006.

Pollan, Michael. *The Omnivore's Dilemma: A Natural History of Four Meals.* New York: Penguin, 2006.

Schlosser, Eric. *Fast Food Nation: The Dark Side of the All-American Meal.* Boston: Houghton Mifflin, 2001.

Shiva, Vandana. *Stolen Harvest: The Hijacking of the Global Food Supply.* Cambridge, MA: South End, 2000.

Smith, Alisa and J. B. Mackinnon. *Plenty: One Man, One Woman, and A Raucous Year of Eating Locally.* New York: Harmony, 2007.

Smith, Edward C. *Incredible Vegetables from Self-Watering Containers.* North Adams, MA: Storey, 2006.

———. *The Vegetable Gardener's Bible.* North Adams, MA: Storey, 2000.

Trubek, Amy B. *The Taste of Place: A Cultural Journey into Terroir.* Berkeley: University of California, 2008.

Vinton, Sherri Brooks and Ann Clark Espuelas. *The Real Food Revival: Aisle by Aisle, Morsel by Morsel.* New York: Penguin, 2005.

Waters, Alice. *The Art of Simple Food: Notes, Lessons and Recipes from a Delicious Revolution.* New York: Clarkson Potter, 2007.

Winne, Mark. *Closing the Food Gap: Resetting the Table in the Land of Plenty.* Boston: Beacon, 2008.

Wirzba, Norman, ed. *The Art of the Commonplace: The Agrarian Essays of Wendell Berry.* Washington, D.C.: Shoemaker & Hoard, 2002.

MOVIES

Beyond Organic: The Vision of Fairview Gardens
Available from Bullfrog Films. Visit their website at: *www.bullfrogfilms.com*

Deconstructing Supper: Is Your Food Safe?
Available from Bullfrog Films. Visit their website at: *www.bullfrogfilms.com*

Food, Inc.
www.foodincmovie.com

King Corn
Independent Lens, PBS
www.pbs.org/independentlens/kingcorn
Information on the film.

The Meatrix Trilogy
For more information, and to watch the films, visit: *www.meatrix.com*

My Father's Garden
Available from Miranda Productions. Visit their website at: *http://mirandaproductions.com*

The Real Dirt on Farmer John
Available from Farmer John Productions, Angelic Organics. Visit their website at: *www.angelicorganics.com*

Two Angry Moms
For more information visit:
www.angrymoms.org

INDEX

G

H

I

J

K

L

M

N

O

P

T

U

V

W

Y

Z

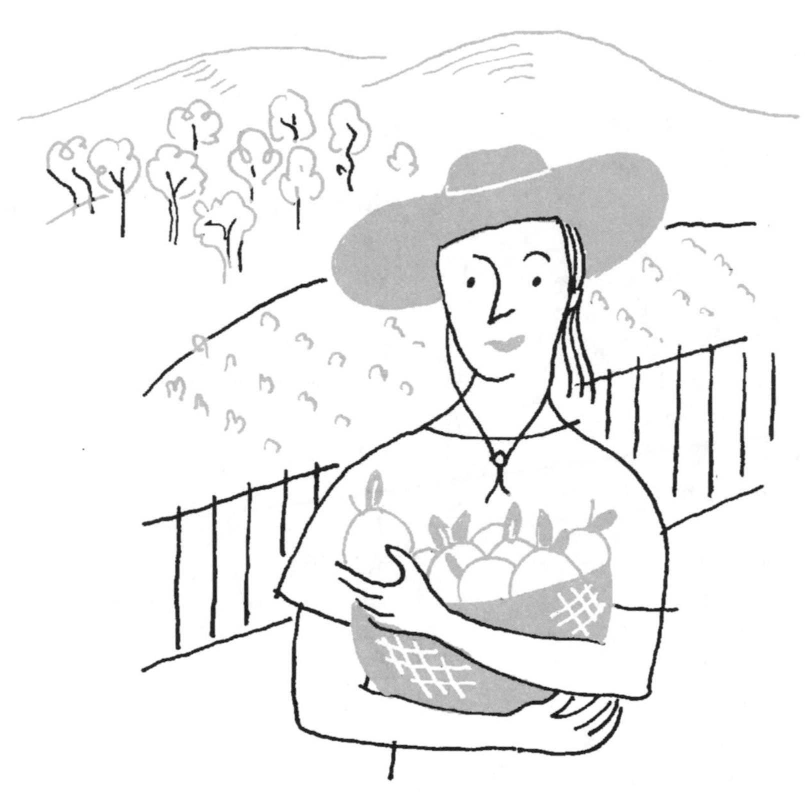

ABOUT THE AUTHOR

A PASSIONATE EATER, culinary professional, and veteran advocate of local eating, Amy Cotler consults, teaches, and lectures on food and farm-to-fork issues. She is the founding director of Berkshire Grown, a small nonprofit that supports local food and farms, which has served as an early model for grassroots organizations here and abroad.

Ms. Cotler has worked in Manhattan and the Berkshires — her home in western Massachusetts — as a chef, caterer, cooking teacher, recipe developer, food writer, and cookbook author. Her five cookbooks include *Wrap it Up* and *Fresh from the Farm: The Massachusetts Farm to School Cookbook*, a tool for schools, which is available free online through her Web site. Her food articles have been published in periodicals, including *Fine Cooking, Kitchen Garden, Cook's, Family Fun, Self, Gastronomica,* and *Orion*. Ms. Cotler has developed close to 1,000 recipes, many of which are featured in the revised *The Joy of Cooking*. She has appeared on The Food Network and National Public Radio and was a longtime food forum host for the *New York Times* on the Web.

A lively teacher and lecturer, Ms. Cotler speaks at diverse venues, from small community-based organizations to colleges, such as Williams and Radcliffe. She taught at the Institute for Culinary Education and The Culinary Institute of America, where she also wrote teaching text for their professional cookbook. She continues to teach and give farm tours regionally and from the country kitchen in her 1810 home. She also initiates and consults on a wide range of local food based projects, such as those boosting farm-fresh food in local schools and connecting regional chefs and farmers.

Ms. Cotler lives with her husband, artist Tom Powers, her daughter, Emma, and their cat, Leroy. A lazy weeder, she has a vegetable garden and likes hosting pot luck suppers. Reach her on her Web site and blog at *www.amycotler.com*.

OTHER STOREY TITLES YOU WILL ENJOY

THE BACKYARD HOMESTEAD, EDITED BY CARLEEN MADIGAN.

A complete guide to growing and raising the most local food available anywhere — from one's own backyard.

352 PAGES. PAPER. ISBN 978-1-60342-138-6.

THE BEGINNER'S GUIDE TO PRESERVING FOOD AT HOME, BY JANET CHADWICK.

The best and quickest methods for preserving every common vegetable and fruit, with easy instructions to encourage even first-timers.

240 PAGES. PAPER. ISBN 978-1-60342-145-4.

PUMPKIN, BY DEEDEE STOVEL.

A wide-ranging collection of recipes, from soups to desserts and everything in between that use this nutritious orange super food.

224 PAGES. PAPER. ISBN 978-1-58017-594-4.

ROOT CELLARING, BY MIKE AND NANCY BUBEL.

Suitable for city and country folks, with information on harvesting and creating cold storage anywhere — even closets! — plus 50 recipes.

320 PAGES. PAPER. ISBN 978-0-88266-703-4.

SERVING UP THE HARVEST, BY ANDREA CHESMAN.

A collection of 175 recipes to bring out the best in garden-fresh vegetables, with 14 master recipes that can accommodate whatever happens to be in your produce basket.

516 PAGES. PAPER. ISBN 978-1-58017-663-7.

These and other books from Storey Publishing are available wherever quality books are sold or by calling 1-800-441-5700. Visit us at www.storey.com.